CRUSADER'S CLINIC

GEORGE SAVA

WILLIAM KIMBER · LONDON

First published in 1977 by
WILLIAM KIMBER & CO. LIMITED
Godolphin House, 22a Queen Anne's Gate,
London, SW1H 9AE

© George Sava, 1977
ISBN 0 7183 0075 0

Filmset by
Specialised Offset Services Limited, Liverpool
and printed and bound in Great Britain by
Redwood Burn Limited, Trowbridge and Esher

CRUSADER'S CLINIC

By the same author:

The Years of the Healing Knife *etc.*

CONTENTS

PROLOGUE

One night, some months ago, I was returning from a medical meeting where the matter of venereal diseases was discussed and the fact stressed that in spite of all the progress made by medical science in the last decade, venereal diseases are on the increase – particularly amongst the younger generation and those with the highest education. Greater sexual permissiveness through the wider use of the pill and the comparative ease of obtaining abortions has meant an increase in the likelihood of VD infection. The words of my friends were still ringing in my ears: 'Why don't you write a book on VD? – Not a treatise or a technical one – those exist by the score – but a book for the average specimen of that widely dispersed variety of homo sapiens, the man-in-the-street. Needless to say, I felt not merely flattered that my friends thought I could write such a book, but instantly fascinated by the idea.

So I began my task – to report facts and facts alone in as palatable and arresting a fashion as was possible so that any inquiring citizen could read and gain more information. And to put those same inquiring citizens at ease, let me point out that it is not only VD which is transmitted through sexual intercourse. Scientists know now that more than twenty-five infectious diseases may and can be transmitted by sexual intercourse. Why then the shame or guilt that many sufferers from VD feel? The answer is simple: ignorance – yes, ignorance, misguided social and religious prejudice and lack of real knowledge of venereal diseases as a whole.

In this book I have tried to dispense with all this. My chief aim is to answer many questions that were and are still puzzling ordinary people. I have also tried to show that while many infectious diseases can be transmitted through sexual intercourse, VD too can be a non-sexual infection. In that case then does VD still enjoy such infamy; why is it still the *enfant terrible* of medicine – at least in the eyes of the general public? There is only one answer: ignorance and social prejudice.

I feel joy and satisfaction in my heart that before I even finished writing this book, new laws and an enlightened approach to the problem of VD have been adopted and even enacted in Parliament. Now the problem becomes mainly a medical one – We have to conquer the disease by purely medical means. That is an unassailable truth. The social and sociological aspect is almost solved through the enlightened public opinion that has already taken the rightful path.

In a democracy such as ours and most of the Western World enlightened opinion can still be furthered by more information, factual information, unbiased information – the sole basis for intelligent judgment.

That is precisely the sort of information I have tried to assemble in my book. Whether I have succeeded or not, only the future can determine. If the inquiring public believes and avows that it is something every one of them should read, if they are ever to begin to think straight on a subject that has for so long lain, like Nature's laws, 'hid in night' though the night, to speak truth, has been and is still more a fog of man's own making; if the book then succeeds in dispersing the fog that is still there, then I have succeeded in my task.

Finally I would like to emphasize as strongly as possible one salient fact which has been introduced for the better understanding of the subject by the layman. Clinics, doctors and patients are real, but their names and locations have been changed for obvious reasons. Yet if by some coincidence, some do correspond to the name of some real person or place, this is purely coincidental and I apologise for any such unwitting similarity.

With this brief prologue, let me introduce *Crusader's Clinic* as a tribute to the untiring work of the medical profession as a whole and to the enlightened layman and woman in general.

GEORGE SAVA

Introducing
Jonathan Miles

Jonathan Miles is a doctor with the usual higher qualifications – that is to say he is an MD, FRCP and DPH. This is by the way of professional introduction. His present appointment is as Director of the Department for the Treatment of Venereal Diseases at the Maynard Clinic; and that is the part of it which is most important.

Today, almost everybody has heard of the Maynard Clinic, the largest and most complete medical establishment of its kind outside the United States of America. Miles's own department was the last to be added to it but that does not make it by any means the least interesting. On the contrary, it is because he felt that the work of this department was so full of cases of the greatest human significance and of something much more than mere medical interest, that I have come to write this book about him.

The steps that led to his making VD his speciality are, in effect, a reflection of a very widespread attitude to this subject and provide an answer to the question that so many people have asked him with a look of pained surprise and a veiled hint of disgust, 'But what on earth, doctor, led you to take up this?'

If he had run true to form, it is certain that he should never have taken the course he did in life. He was brought up in a typical middle class atmosphere, where it was not considered decent to notice unpleasant truths and the comfortable belief was held that by ignoring a thing it ceased to exist. That was the general atmosphere; his own home was one in which it was carried to the point of suffocation.

He often wondered what the effect would have been if anyone had so much as whispered the words 'venereal disease' in his father's presence; for him, of course, as for the majority of people at that time, VD would have been regarded as the punishment for sin; and some even held the extreme opinion that a doctor who tried to cure it shared in his patient's sin and flew in the face of Providence, to use one of their favourite phrases.

So it cannot be said that Jonathan began to specialize in the subject because he had been brought up by enlightened teachers thirsting for social reform; the exact contrary was the truth.

During Jonathan Miles's training, venereal diseases were greatly on the increase and he had to come up against them, but he was at a small provincial university where old conventions died hard. It is rather curious that the hold of old ideas was so strong on Miles that even though he tried to be coldly scientific, he never quite lost a belief that there was something different about VD – something that put it apart from other diseases, something that called for a special approach; he was certainly not alone in this. Patients who came to the hospital for VD treatment were, of course, treated in secrecy, with only numbers on their cards for identification. There was something furtive about the whole business. Even the doctors in charge of the cases gave the impression that they would much rather be on other work; and indeed, there was a tendency to allocate to VD wards house physicians and house surgeons who had not shown up too brightly elsewhere.

When Miles qualified, he was in exactly the same state as every other fledgeling doctor, which means that he knew a little about very many things but practically nothing complete about any one of them. Any idea of specialization, whether in VD or anything else, never crossed his mind. His only thought was to get as much experience as possible and to that extent at least his subsequent interest was almost the result of an accident.

Two incidents, he would tell you, stand out vividly in his mind when he tries to recall what it was that led him to his speciality. These were I think, the real starting points, the personal experiences that led him to devote whatever power and talents he possessed to fighting this scourge.

The first happened about a year after Jonathan had qualified and he was working in a small hospital in the North of England. He had to assist a pathologist making a couple of post mortems, one on a man in his early fifties, the other on a younger man of about thirty. Both had died suddenly and for reasons best known to himself, the coroner had decided that autopsies should be made, though in each case the case of death seemed obvious enough. The man of fifty had died of advanced untreated syphilis, the other from TB.

Miles had never seen a post mortem on either condition before and with his still biased way of thinking he not unnaturally expected to find that the internal degeneration of the syphilis would be far greater than that of the TB patient. He still thought that syphilis was like some terrible thing gnawing its victim to death.

In actual fact, that state of affairs was entirely the opposite. This is not the place to enter into great medical detail and I will say no more than that the internal condition of a person who has died from syphilis is not infrequently less revolting than in cases of diseases generally regarded as 'normal'.

So much for the first of these incidents. Some years later, Jonathan moved to a larger and more modern hospital in the West of England which was one of the comparatively few with a VD department. He asked the Medical Superintendent for a chance of working in that section, not because he had any special desire to study VD deeply, but simply because he was eager for new experience. A few days later he was told by the physician in charge of the VD department that he would work with him.

Dr Ames, as I shall call him, had a rather grim sense of humour. He decided that Miles' enthusiasm had better be put at once to a test of sincerity. He took him to a small ward containing a single bed but he paused before allowing him to see the patient.

'This patient,' he said, 'is a three years old girl and she has delayed syphilis, showing all the advanced signs of tertiary degeneration. Her father died in this hospital of General Paralysis of the Insane (known by its initial letters GPI) a year ago and her mother is still under treatment. The poor child has done nothing herself, except choosing the wrong parents. Now you can look at her!'

Jonathan did so. 'Even with all I have seen since', he will tell you, 'I do not think I have ever come across a more terrible example of what used to be called hereditary syphilis.' The child seemed to his inexperienced eyes, barely human. Its physical condition was shocking enough but even more appalling was its utter lack of any spark of human intelligence. It barely possessed so much as the power of animal movements. It was a ghastly travesty of a living creature.

Dr Ames looked at the young doctor with a slight shrug.

'The best and the most hopeful thing I can say about this case,' he said, 'is that she cannot live much longer. The grimmest thought of all,' he added, 'is that if she were an animal and I a vet, I could end that tragedy. But she is a human being. Therefore she must live to the last moment.'

It is not difficult to picture the intense horror with which Jonathan Miles was filled. Partly, that reaction came from the sight of the tragic child herself, but partly too, it was transmitted from Dr Ames himself. And to this day the feeling of intense pity and disgust which Dr Ames betrayed at the time, remains with Miles, whenever a syphilitic child is brought to him for treatment. It has nothing to do with the tragic little patient, but is an indignation against a society that allows such things to continue and, more than that, puts barriers in the path of those stricken down by its own gross stupidity.

It was a revolution of feeling that many people would have had in those circumstances, to resolve to devote themselves to the cure of VD, but resolutions so made are more often broken than kept. It was the quiet persistent encouragement of Dr Ames that made Miles see that he had the right qualifications for specializing in VD work. It was he who finally eradicated the last shreds of his moral aversion and made him see the whole problem as one entirely for medicine and its allied sciences.

I do not think that I have seen in my own practice, any case worse than that which Dr Ames introduced to the young Jonathan Miles at the time.

It is because of these and a hundred other things like them that I have written this book about this dedicated man, Jonathan Miles. It is intended to be another weapon in the fight against not only a terrible disease but also the fear and prejudice which causes hundreds of people to suffer every year for sins they have never committed, or just as pathetic – they chose to suffer in silence because of the shame in which venereal diseases are still shrouded in this enlightened day. We have got to recognize the fact that the knowledge which medical research discovers and which now has been made freely available to all in the interests of fuller, happier and healthier lives must be fully explained. The theme of this book is that the venereal diseases are in no way different from any of the others. They provide a medical problem and a scientific one and the question of morals comes into them only incidentally. That is a conviction of a lifetime and every new case I chance to see confirms it.

The first three cases are from my own case-book. All those following are from Jonathan Miles's. I was fortunate enough to have gained permission from him to present his case-histories and comments as he gave them to me, and for the sake of continuity and easy reading I have kept his cases in the first person.

Case 1

MARILYN

I shall always remember Marilyn with affection and gratitude. Affection because she is a charming, unassuming young lady, the daughter of a patient of mine; and gratitude because providence sent her to me when she was most in need of help and comfort.

I first met Marilyn as a teenager. A lanky youngster, all legs and arms at the time, she was with her mother who had come to consult me at my Harley Street rooms. Mrs Smith, (not her real name), was a widowed school teacher of about forty years of age. They came from Lancashire – a county which holds a special place in my heart. It was in Lancashire that I started my English career as a surgeon. Mrs Smith came to consult me for an undiagnosed abdominal pain. I was quick to recognise an acute appendicitis and was able to operate on her almost immediately. She recovered very quickly and in no time was able to resume teaching in Manchester.

They had come to London because Mrs Smith wanted me to operate on her and because her sister – also an old patient of mine – lived in Hampstead. Thus she could convalesce there and be with her sister whom she had not visited for a long time. Marilyn, a girl of about thirteen years of age and already showing signs of future beauty, stayed with her mother and aunt and as I visited them practically every day, we became fast friends and I grew to adore the little girl.

That was some years ago and although we did not see each other again, the mother kept informing me about Marilyn's progress at school. I was overjoyed to hear that Marilyn had passed her teacher's exams with honour and was now on her first teaching job at the same school at which her mother was employed. For two years Marilyn worked hard and saved every penny she could. One of her great dreams was to go on a long and extensive visit to Paris. A postcard from Dover informed me that her dream was about to be realised. It was her first real holiday and she was going to enjoy it to the full. Knowing her mother and the strict but very loving upbringing she had received from her, I had no qualms about her going to Paris. After all, she was now twenty-one years of age, spoke French and was in the company with two other girls. She had given me the name of the hotel in Paris and I promptly wrote her a card wishing her a really enjoyable time. After that, work compelled me to put Marilyn and other holidaying friends out of my mind.

But I was sorely mistaken in thinking that Marilyn was going to have just a pleasant holiday, after which she would resume her former life. Her mother's frantic call one evening at my home upset me greatly. In a broken voice – I was sure that she was crying on the other side of the line – she informed me that Marilyn was not returning to England.

'Why, what's the matter?' I asked. 'She's not ill, is she? And surely – not an accident?'

'No, she is not ill, but you might well call it a terrible accident!'

'Then she is hurt!'

'No, not in the physical sense, but something has happened to my girl that frightens me to death.'

'Please, Mrs Smith, calm yourself and tell me what's really the matter.'

The story I now heard was certainly a terrible one from a mother's point of view, but to me it was far from tragic. Marilyn had fallen in love with a young Frenchman whom she had met on an outing to the Louvre Galleries. Apparently it was love – a mutual one – at first sight. The girl had simply fallen head over heels in love. She had resigned her job at the school in England and was going to stay in Paris with the man she loved.

I tried to calm her mother saying that after all Frenchmen, as a rule, are good husbands and she must not be too English minded in thinking that only Englishmen are worth marrying.

'I wouldn't mind him being a foreigner but the fact is that they don't plan to marry at all! They just want to live together for a while to see if they are suited to each other.'

'Well, even that's not as bad as it sounds, Mrs Smith,' I tried to console the frantic mother. 'Nowadays young people are very liberated in their outlook and I'm sure it will all work itself out. Please don't upset yourself unnecessarily. I suggest you go and see for yourself. After all, Marilyn is a level-headed, educated girl and I'm sure she knows what is she doing. Once you've met him you might see things differently.'

'No, I don't want to see them!' came the curt reply. There was such bitterness and pain in her voice that even at a distance I could sense that so far as she was concerned, her daughter had transgressed beyond redemption.

I tried in vain to reason with Mrs Smith. I tried in vain to comfort and calm her. It is not so much that I myself, approve of all things modern and liberated or progressive. But I do realise that not all of it is bad and much of it begins to make good sense when considered without prejudice and above all with 'cool'. After all would it be not far better to live together for a while and discover if a young couple are suited to each other or not, than to have a hasty marriage which ends in the divorce courts. So once again I had to dismiss Marilyn from my mind sincerely hoping that her mother would eventually see the light and all three become somewhat reconciled to their delicate relationship.

For three months I did not hear from either of them – both mother and daughter obviously had decided to keep their troubles to themselves. The next time, however, I heard from them it was in my consulting rooms. This time it was Marilyn herself who came to see me – without an appointment. One glance at that still beautiful but drawn and haggard face was enough to convince me that some terrible tragedy had struck her. I did not press her for the reason for her visit, but welcomed her as gently and as casually as I could, giving her time to tell me her story when she felt ready and uninhibited enough to do so.

Marilyn apologised for her unorthodox intrusion. As it happened it was practically five in the afternoon – the closing hour for consultations. She wanted to say something, her lips moved but no sound came. Then she simply burst into heart-rending sobs which all this time she must have tried to suppress.

'Marilyn,' I said, putting my arm round her shoulder. 'My secretary wants to lock up here. Perhaps it would be better if I took you along home with me. You look very tired and before you tell me about your troubles, you'd best rest a while and have a meal. I've a feeling you haven't eaten a bite today.'

She did not speak but simply nodded in agreement. Slowly I led her to the street where my car was parked and in no time we were sitting in the lounge while a hot bowl of soup was being prepared for her in the kitchen. At my express bidding we were left alone and gradually her tale began to unfold.

It really was a sad story, to say the least. Yes, she had fallen in love with the young Frenchman and gone to live with him in his apartment somewhere on the Left Bank. It was, at first, every young girl's dream of love come true. Never had she known such happiness.

That happiness lasted, however, for only about a month. One day Marilyn felt sick and feverish. François had already gone to work and she was alone. She felt so sick and frightened that she realised she must get hold of a doctor. In desperation she searched the telephone directory for a doctor's address. Fortunately there was one – a GP almost opposite their apartment. So Marilyn phoned him saying that she felt very ill and could she come to see him as soon as possible. The answer was naturally 'Yes'.

The doctor examined her carefully, noticing particularly the many red spots all over her body. He wanted to know how long she had had these spots, but Marilyn did not know. She had noticed them only that morning when she tried to take her temperature.

Without saying anything further the doctor wrote a note and told her to go to a particular hospital not too distant from where she lived. He gave her the exact address. When she stepped out of her taxi, Marilyn found herself in the out-patients department of a rather grimy and very dilapidated building. The nurse took her particulars and soon an elderly doctor came and examined her carefully. Samples of urine and blood were taken, some kind of tablets for the fever were given and Marilyn was told to return in two days' time.

That evening she told François her distressing day. To her surprise he showed her remarkably little sympathy. Upon her return to the hospital she was at once taken to another department and asked to wait. Soon another doctor came and without any preliminaries, he informed her that she was suffering from syphilis – first acute stage – and that she must receive treatment at once. They told her that she must come daily for shots and must have no intercourse with anyone.

For a while Marilyn stood there uncomprehending and totally bewildered. 'But, Doctor,' she managed to say. 'This is impossible! There must be some ghastly mistake. I have never had any sexual relations with anybody except – my husband.'

She called him her husband because she thought of him as her husband and at that time he was her husband. She explained to me that her deception was not intentional. She really considered him as her husband – if not in law at least in spirit.

Of course there was no mistake. She had at least three different tests and all of them were positive. On further examination – causing great distress and embarrassment to Marilyn – she was forced to undergo gynaecological examination and that too revealed the primary minute ulcer on her genital organs – the contact and entrance of the virulent spirochaeta. The syphilitic microbe had done its ugly work and the red spots on Marilyn's body were evidence that the disease had already spread all over her body and contaminated her blood.

She was given a shot, then handed a card with the terse reminder to attend the clinic daily or if she wished, and was able to pay, she could be admitted as an in-patient. Marilyn fled from the hospital and still unbelieving waited for her boyfriend to return from work. Surely he would tell her that this could not be true and reassure her that all would be well. At any rate he would take care of her. After all, nothing could come between a love like theirs.

When François eventually came home the help and

understanding she expected from him was conspicuously absent. On the contrary, he assumed an outraged, insulted, almost arrogant air and accused her of being unfaithful to him. When Marilyn protested and burst out crying, instead of the sympathy she so yearned for, she received more insults.

'You English slut, you go around with anybody and try to pin it on me? Thank God,' he lied unashamedly, 'thank God I used a condom (a protective sheet) so at least you couldn't give the syphilis to me. You're just a bloody tart! Get out of my home and don't you dare come back!'

And so he threw her out. And that was about eight in the evening. Marilyn left the apartment and as she told me, in her desperation she stood for hours near the river thinking that the best way out of all this nightmare, was the soft oblivion of the Seine's muddy waters.

I am sure she would have killed herself, but for her sound English – North English – background and the love she had for her mother. Shedding unrestrained tears, she told me that when she almost was ready to jump in the river, the image of her loving mother came vividly to her mind. She realised that by killing herself she would no doubt kill her mother as well. So instead of jumping into the river, Marilyn walked for hours until she reached the Gare du Nord. There, at ten in the morning, she boarded the train and that evening she came to me – she did not know where to go, she told me, and she could not face her mother. Not yet.

That very night I arranged for Marilyn to see Jonathan Miles, the VD specialist. Marilyn stayed in London for a month and received daily treatment. Then she was told to return in three months for another course of treatment. And so for a year young Marilyn continued the treatment and finally she was declared cured.

What of her mother? At the beginning Marilyn begged me not to tell her mother, but I insisted that she must tell her herself. After all these two women loved each other – had once had a perfect relationship. Surely this strong bond had not been entirely severed. Finally I persuaded Marilyn to phone her mother and tell her that she was in London still ill but much better and under my care.

The very next morning her mother was in my consulting rooms. I told her as gently and as delicately as possible the trouble Marilyn was in. While I spoke her mother cried silently but not one word of reproach came forth from her lips. She had always loved her daughter dearly, and now, in her great need, she loved her even more. For suddenly, her grown, independent daughter had become a child again, in need of her care, in dire need of her love.

I am glad to be able to conclude this tragic story with a very enjoyable and happy ending. Yes, Marilyn was cured completely – that is, she was cured physically. Mentally it took longer for the wound to heal. But in the end even that was healed. Three years later, a smiling and happy Marilyn walked again unannounced into my rooms – this time to present her fiance to me. At my slightly enquiring look, she smiled and told me that John knew all about her former troubles. 'You cannot be happy with a man if your life is based on a lie,' she said in deadly earnest. John was a man of understanding. He loved Marilyn as much as she loved him. They both insisted on final tests, because they wanted children and wanted to be sure that nothing would impair their children's health. Again my VD specialist friend took the tests personally. Now Marilyn and John – both teachers somewhere in England – are enjoying a happy life with their two children and all four share the devotion of Mrs Smith who lives with them.

'She's an unbelievably good grandmother!' they both told me. So a sickening tragedy was transformed; little by little it was entirely erased and a new, healthy and useful life built on its site.

THE TWO FRIENDS

Every time I think of those two young friends and the circumstances that brought them to my professional attention, I cannot help experiencing some kind of frustration as well as gratitude that providence more than professional help, turned an almost inevitable tragedy into a routine treatment for a disease which nearly ruined both their young lives.

Steven and Arnold were friends from early childhood. Steven's background was very proper, typical middle-class English; his father was a solicitor. The boy was just ten years of age when they moved to their new house. He was a shy, rather retiring boy who did not make friends easily. He was, however, brilliant at school and that brought him to the attention of the older boy. Arnold – Arny to his friends – liked the new boy and immediately appointed himself his protector. And which shy, new school-boy does not welcome a friend when faced with the inevitable pranks and snide remarks that plague all new school-children.

So Steven was grateful to Arny for his protection and in return gave him the unstinted devotion which was to last all their schooldays. It is rather surprising that these two boys became such inseparable friends. Surprising because of their utterly different backgrounds.

Steven's family life, so very conservative, was nevertheless close and devoted. He had a younger brother and a baby sister – all dearly loved by their parents. It was not in their nature to let love gain the upper hand and their idea of upbringing was thus strict with not even a hint of spoiling or endulging.

On the other hand Arnold's family background was one all too familiar in this day and age – that of broken marriage.

Arnold was only five years of age when his mother left and he was to see very little of her from that day. Soon there was a stepmother, however, a good wife perhaps, but not a loving stepmother. That marriage was also doomed and Arnold at his twelfth birthday was presented with yet another stepmother.

When these two boys became friends, Steven was ten and Arnold three years his senior. It is rather surprising that Steven's father who obviously knew of the other boy's family background and most likely disapproved, did not prevent his son's friendship with this older boy. Perhaps he realised that the child's devotion to his friend was too great to destroy. Steven's mother although frequently unhappy at the thought of this strange friendship must also have felt that to put a stop to it might prove even more harmful. But she could not hide her distaste when Steven, in his innocence, occasionally related the adventures of his older friend. 'You know, Mummy, Arny tells me that he often sleeps with his cousin Susie when she stays at their house.' Steven's mother would feign some kind of amusement and tell her son that perhaps Arnold was frightened of the dark, since he had no brothers or sisters. Of course she hardly thought for a moment that the intelligent boy would believe her. Still what was she to do? She hoped with all her heart that his good upbringing, his love for his family and above all his intelligence, would keep him from harm. And so the two boys' friendship thrived undisturbed for some years.

I personally never met Arnold, that is, not until the time of the tragedy. But I had met Steven and his parents. It was his congenital – inborn – hernia that brought Steven to my rooms. The boy was rather fond of sports and the school doctor on a routine examination, had found that Steven was suffering from a mild degree of inguinal hernia. In other circumstances this would not have required an operation, but Steven was taking part in school Rugby and High Jump and the doctor thought that the boy might get the small hernia strangulated from the exertion. So on his advice Steven was brought to my consulting rooms for examination. I agreed with the doctor's diagnosis and advised an operation. In the summer holidays

Steven was operated on, recovered well and the following year won prize in sport – high jumping.

Occasionally I was told by his father of his son's progress – we belonged to the same social club and whenever we met I always enquired about Steven. The answer was always the same: Steven was very healthy and very good in both his studies and his sport-activities. So some years passed – four to be exact – until I again heard from Steven. This time it was the boy, now a seventeen years old teenager, who came to see me. He had made an appointment but the name did not ring a bell when I saw it on the list of the day's patients.

I was terribly surprised when I did eventually realise who my patient was. Not because it was Steven, but because of the way he looked and walked. It was obvious that the boy was in terrible pain and could scarcely walk.

'Doctor,' he pleaded, 'please help me! I can't stand it any more!'

I did not ask many questions excepting the necessary ones such as how the illness began and where exactly it hurt. As Steven replied, my suspicions were instantly aroused. I needed only a short examination to confirm those supicions. Yes, Steven was suffering from an acute disease – most likely from gonorrhoea. The discharge – a yellow thick smear that was visible at the end of his urethra and the swollen and extremely painful testicles told their unmistakable tale. Steven was remarkably frank and helpful. The story he had to tell was one only too common today.

Unfortunately young people rarely realise that permissiveness, though outwardly so attractive, like a snake has many hidden hazards. And so it had all begun in fun as it always does. Steven had met his old friend Arny about a week before he came to see me. It was an unexpected and pleasant meeting between two old friends. It was a Saturday and Arny had suggested dinner in Soho and then a movie. The two young men had laughed and joked a great deal. But when Steven suggested it was time to go home, Arny had smiled mysteriously and said he still had a surprise for Steven. It was a surprise indeed, more than Steven had ever expected or bargained for. Arny said nonchalantly that they were going to visit some friends of his he was sure Steven would like. It turned out that the visit was at a shabby flat occupied by two young girls – personal friends of Arny's.

Steven was not exactly pleased with the visit, but being a polite boy he decided not to say anything and stayed on with his friend. After all there was no harm having a drink or two with Arny's friends. These two drinks, however, led to more and yet more – the sort of binge only a hardened drinker can master. Steven was not quite clear as to what happened after that. As I understood it, the boy ended up in bed with one of the girls and was initiated in the art of sex. Embarrassed or ashamed of his adventures, he naturally did not tell his mother about it.

Two days later, however, he was awaken by a searing pain when trying to urinate and he noticed that his testicles were very swollen and red. He grew frantic with fear particularly of his very strict father. In despair he thought of me. Although it was over four years since the operation on his hernia he obviously could not think of a single person other than myself, to whom he dared disclose his tale of woe.

Laboratory tests confirmed my provisional diagnosis. It was gonorrhoea and in its most virulent form. As a rule the disease affects only the urethral canal and only if not treated properly does it affect the bladder and the testicles. In Steven's case it had taken the most virulent form. Both his bladder and testicles were infected and there was the danger of an abscess and complete ruin of the boy's future sex life.

There was no time to lose. I personally made an appointment with Jonathan Miles and drove Steven to the clinic. Fortunately for all of us, particularly for Steven, he was not living at home by that time. These were his long summer holidays and he had taken a job in the city. Wishing to be near his work and also to gain more independence, he had found himself a bachelor flat. So his parents were kept at a safe distance from their son and his unfortunate predicament – for the present, that is. His father's reaction, I suspected, would be anything but sympathetic and that in itself would only have worsened his son's condition.

An immediate and vigorous treatment was instituted and

on the insistence of my friend, Steven was admitted to hospital for a few days, because of the danger that the complication might turn into an abscess of the testicles necessitating an operation. Fortunately this did not occur. In a few days the swelling and pain subsided and Steven was released from the hospital and went home to his flat. In the meantime I had informed his temporary employers that Steven was not well and would be absent from work. Thus there would be no give-away questions at his parents' home.

For all the summer holidays Steven received regular treatment for gonorrhoea and before the vacation was over, he was declared perfectly cured. When Steven returned to his own home he was his former self and began his last year at school, preparing for his A level exams and entry in Law at London University – the school where his own father had studied. All the treatment was kept completely secret and even the name was altered so that no identification could be made by enquiring busybodies. I do not know whether Steven ever told his parents about his mishap. I certainly did not ask him. That was his own affair. I was glad that he was cured and knowing him as I do, I feel convinced that sooner or later he will confess his 'guilt' to his understanding mother at least. But in actual fact there is no need now for him to tell anyone since he is considered clear.

The case of the other protagonist of the drama – Arny – was quite another thing. By a freak of nature, the disease in Arnold did not take the violent course that it had in Steven. With the exception of some mild pain while urinating and a slight continuous discharge from his urethra, Arnold did not suffer anything more; not for the time being, anyway. But whereas his body suffered so little, here it was the mind that was affected. And this took quite a dreadful turn. Perhaps it was the fault of his unhappy childhood – his mother deserting him; the two step-mothers who were not exactly loving mothers. All these facts must have taken root in the boy's mind and begun to turn him against women. Then the episode with the girl and his infection and what were already misgivings soon must have turned to genuine hate and antagonism against all women and fast ones in particular.

I asked Steven to contact his friend and persuade him either to see me or to go to a VD clinic. Nothing happened, however. Arny would not hear of it. He was bent up on revenge and apparently went in search of young girls – not so much for sex as to give them a dose of what they had given him. Arny was young and very attractive to women, particularly teenagers and school-girls. God knows what would have happened if no measures had been taken to prevent his escapades. How many trusting but fun-loving girls would have ended up in VD clinics or had their entire adult lives ruined. Gonorrhoea is even more dangerous in women than in men. Even when treated, the woman may end up with permanent sterility because of the Fallopian tubes of her uterus being affected and closed permanently, so that no sperms or eggs can pass through them.

It was obvious to me that Arny must be induced to undergo treatment as soon as possible so as to prevent him from spreading the disease to others and for his own sake as well. One can understand the young man's desire for revenge; but then nobody asked him to go to the flat of his 'friends' and have sex with them in the first place. Perhaps those two girls did not even know themselves that they were infected. It was also imperative to trace them as well and force them to undergo the treatment. I was at a loss as to what to do for the best, so I went to see Jonathan Miles and told him what Steven had related to me about the original culprits and Arny's desire for 'revenge'.

'We have to stop that, my friend,' he said with a frown. 'Do you know the boy's address?' he demanded. 'And the address of the two girls responsible for the boy's infection?'

As a matter of fact Steven had already given both the address of the girls and of Arny's whereabout. So I could say 'Yes' to Jonathan's demand.

'That's splendid,' he said. 'I'll go and see the blighter myself.'

'But can you force him and the girls to go to the clinic?'

'Oh yes, I can. I'll call the police if necessary.'

There was no need for the police or the special branch that deals with VD carriers. What Jonathan had said to Arny or with what he had threatened him I never was to know. The truth is that the very day he saw Arnold, the young man was already on his way to the clinic. As a matter of fact, it was Jonathan who took Arny to his clinic and began the treatment at once. As to the two girls the moment they were told that they had been suffering from gonorrhoea, they more than willingly agreed to be treated.

Arny was also induced to name all of the girls he had slept with after that night at the flat of the two infected women. Once he was assured that nothing would happen to the girls and that their parents would not find out, Arny revealed the names of three very respectable young school-girls. These were gently and diplomatically approached by women VD sleuths and told that they might be infected with a very serious disease that could ruin their lives if not treated immediately and properly. They were assured that their parents would not be informed. The girls were examined. All three showed signs of gonorrhoea. Immediate treatment was instituted and by the end of the summer holidays they all three resumed their studies healthy and perhaps the wiser for the unpleasant escapades which could have turned into real tragedies.

So one way or the other, the two young friends were cured from the disease. They remained friends, but I doubt if they ever visited any more casual friends. I am convinced that both Steven and Arnold took their sex-lives a great deal more seriously after their harrowing experiences. Nothing can be more off-putting to promiscuity than the threat of VD – especially to someone who has already experienced the disease in all its unpleasant forms.

Case 3

THE CHANCE ENCOUNTER

When I first saw Magda – an attractive woman in her early thirties, I never thought that she would end up becoming a patient and later ask for my help in a quite unexpected and bizarre situation. For I met Magda socially (her surname is omitted) at a cocktail party given by a friend of mine, a very successful City publicity man. Both he and his wife were running an advertising agency and because of their work they often entertained at their home. I met them by chance and we immediately struck up a friendship. So I was not surprised to receive an invitation to attend their next cocktail and dinner party.

It was a sumptuous affair and I enjoyed it immensely. Then, while sipping my favourite Manhattan cocktail, I was introduced to a late arrival, a young woman named Magda. Perhaps she was of foreign origin – Hungarian – but her flawless English betrayed nothing foreign; impeccable Oxford English. She was delightful and full of charm. We chatted on casual subjects ranging from politics to the plight of the English economy. Later on, she came up to talk to me again.

'I'm told you're a fabulous plastic surgeon,' she flattered me unashamedly.

'I don't know about the "fabulous" but I'm a plastic surgeon, yes.'

'Modesty doesn't become you, doctor,' she smiled frivolously. 'Our hosts speak of you in glowing terms.'

'They exaggerate, as usual – as all friends do. Besides they're in the advertising business and cannot get out of the habit of extolling their merchandise.' We both laughed and took another glass from the passing waiter's tray.

'One of these days I'll consult you professionally,' were Magda's passing words as we shook hands.

To be truthful I never expected to see Magda again, certainly not as a patient. But I was wrong. Hardly two weeks passed when my secretary informed me that a patient wanted to see me. 'That's all right,' I answered. 'Give her an appointment.'

'I tried, but the lady insists on seeing you after the usual hours. As a matter of fact, she wants to come after five this afternoon.'

I glanced at my appointment book. There was nothing in it for the evening and since as a rule I dined at home late, I thought I might accommodate the lady. After all, ladies were unpredictable. I did not even bother to find out her name. 'Let her come,' I told my secretary, 'and then you needn't wait for her departure. I'll see her out after the consultation.'

I am never surprised at the unusual requests some patients demand, particularly women. My work is mainly plastic surgery and some women do not like to be seen by other patients. That is why I never refuse to accommodate such patients. The surprise, therefore, was not so much her late coming as the identity of the patient herself. It was no other but my casual acquaintance at the cocktail party. The delightful Magda – full of charm and wit, as usual. We chatted for a while, reminiscing about our mutual hosts and their parties.

'You didn't take me seriously when I told you that one day I might consult you professionally, did you?'

'No, I didn't,' I confessed. 'Not because I didn't believe you but I could not see anything in your beautiful face that I could even remotely improve.'

'Perhaps not my face – not yet, anyhow,' she smiled, 'but you haven't seen the rest of me.'

'Oh, I see. And what part of your body do you wish me to see?' I returned the frivolity. 'I mean professionally, what part of yourself do you wish me to examine?'

'My breasts,' she confessed frankly. 'They are rather on the smallish side and I hear that surgeons can do wonders these days with small breasts. Is that true?'

'Yes,' I replied. 'But let me examine you before I give you my opinion.'

I did examine her and I did agree that her breasts were rather small in comparison to the rest of her delightful, sensuous body. I explained in details what could be done and the method to employ. The size of the breasts she left to my judgment. 'You're an expert and you know best. Certainly I do not wish to be stranded with breasts à la Jane Russell.'

Again that infectious laugh that was so exclusively Magda's.

We agreed on the size, on the clinic and on the date of the operation. She was to come to the clinic the following day and I was to operate on her the morning after.

As a rule, particularly in England, for such a minor operation – it takes no more than an hour – and does not entail any danger for a healthy patient. There is no need to go through all the lab tests which are standard in major interventions. I was inclined just to test her urine, take her blood pressure and listen to her heart. But when I enquired about her married life and children, she suddenly informed me that although they were happily married and her husband was very good to her, their happiness was spoiled somewhat by their inability to have children.

'Why?' I asked. 'Is your husband sterile, or is there anything wrong with you?'

'Apparently not. As a matter of fact, I do conceive easily – three times to be exact, since we've been married. But I cannot carry the pregnancy, I always miscarry round about the second or the third month.'

I did not pursue the matter any further, because that was not in my province of specialty. No doubt they had consulted gynaecologists. One thing I did do, however. I decided for no apparent reason to take a sample of her blood. Perhaps it was my American training. I had been working in the USA for some years and there it is law to take amongst the routine lab. tests sample of blood as well, no matter how minor the operation.

I don't claim to have had any premonitions or forbodings. Purely a matter of habit, I suppose, I told her what I intended to do and she readily agreed. 'Don't take too much blood,' she teased. 'I have very little to spare as I have been on a diet for slimming.'

I withdrew from Magda's vein the usual few cc of blood and sent it to the hospital laboratory. The result – a normal one for haemoglobin; the blood corpuscles' count would come in a few days time. In the meantime I operated on Magda and gave her the breasts she wanted. She seemed very pleased with the result and the progress was uneventful. I was on the point of releasing her from the clinic on the third day. On my way to the clinic, I took with me the mail that had arrived that morning.

The letter from the lab, with the result of Magda's blood test I almost replaced in my pocket unopened, but curiosity made me open it. For a moment I could not believe my eyes. 'All tests for VD, even the most sophisticated, were positive.' The older ones were doubtful in their results, so the pathologist had employed the latest and most sensitive test and the result was positive. But he wanted another sample of blood. To be doubly sure. 'Sometimes mistakes had been made for inexplicable reasons,' the letter concluded.

I was truly at a loss as to how best to approach my patient and or what to tell her. I decided on a white lie for the time being. I still hoped that it might be a lab error. I told Magda that she could go home late in the afternoon and come to see me at my rooms for a check-up and for removal of the few stitches. She smiled and said she would. She also agreed to let me take another sample of blood because I told her that they had broken the tube by mistake.

I don't know whether she believed me. Because, as a rule, I am a bad liar and am discovered all too easily. But Magda said nothing, not even a joke about taking too much blood this time. In silence I drew out the necessary amount, smiled at her and bade her good-bye. 'See you next Monday,' I said in parting and left the clinic hurriedly straight for the lab. I left the blood sample and asked to be informed by phone as soon as the tests were through.

The next day the pathologist himself rang me up and told me there was no mistake. Again the tests were positive. There was no doubt Magda was suffering from syphilis in a stage that was not infectious to others but very dangerous to herself. Something had to be done, but what and how?

In America the doctor is bound by law to inform the health authorities and the patient is forced to undergo treatment. Here, in England, the law is not so strict but if only thanks to his conscience, a doctor cannot simply leave a patient untreated even if the disease is not transmittable. Only then did I understand the reason for Magda's repeated miscarriages. It was obviously connected with the disease. I had to talk to her. Knowing what she was – an educated and highly-intelligent woman, I decided not to beat around the bush any longer, but to tell her honestly yet reassuringly that she could be cured even at that late stage.

As it turned out, I was not mistaken in my high opinion of her character. She listened in silence, slightly blushing, but did not interrupt me. I did not ask for confessions. It was not my business. My task was to help her in her predicament and to see that her husband was also examined and treated if necessary. The confession came voluntarily. I told her that it was not necessary for her to tell me anything but she insisted.

'That is the price I am paying for my indiscretion a few months before I was married.' She paused. 'I was already engaged to Robert but decided to have my last fling as a free woman and went to Spain for a holiday.' She continued, 'There were many parties and many so-called Latin lovers. One drink led to another and I found myself dancing with a young gigolo and finished up in my hotel room with him as my bed-partner.'

She apparently noticed that something was wrong when she detected a painful little sore on her genitals. She went to see a doctor. He told her that it was nothing but gave her a few shots of penicillin. She did not know how many, but after the second injection the sore disappeared and when she left Spain the doctor assured her that she had nothing to worry about.

Naturally Magda believed the doctor. It was a pity, because as she said to me, had she doubted the doctor's words or been warned that it might by syphilis, she would have rushed to an English doctor or a clinic to have another check-up and treatment if necessary. But that was three years ago. Now we were faced with the problem of treatment. She gladly consented to see Jonathan Miles. So far so good. But what were we to do with her husband? How could we be sure if he was immune enough to have been left uninfected?

Magda said she would think it over, but in the meantime she began treatment.

I am glad to report that all went well. Magda was cured completely and all the examinations revealed no damage to any of her internal organs or brain tissue. She went further. She loved and respected her husband. She could not live with him, taunted by the knowledge of her escapade and disease. She could not risk his having been unsuspectingly infected. She could not do that to the man she loved.

So Magda decided on a bold move. She would confess her guilt to Robert and if he wished for a divorce she would give it to him even if it would break her heart.

She was right in confessing to her husband, but she was wrong in thinking that he would be unforgiving. Quite the contrary, if anything he became more attentive and sympathetic.. 'Poor girl,' he said. 'Why did you not tell me before? Couldn't you trust me that much?'

The day following her confession they both came to see me and I this time took a sample of his blood. And fate was kind. The repeated tests were all negative. Robert was not infected. The treatment which the Spanish doctor had given Magda had not been complete and could have damaged her body irretrievably. But it did have one advantage. Magda, although not cured herself, was no longer danger to others.

There is an even happier twist to the end of this little story. Six months after the treatment was completed and Magda declared cured, she became pregnant again. In spite of her misgivings and fears, under the expert handling of a fine gynaecologist who was informed of her past history, she kept the pregnancy. Because of her age it was decided that she must be delivered by Caesarian Section. To that both wife and husband agreed and now they enjoy all of the blessings of the happy parents of a baby girl.

At the time of writing, little Magdalena was exactly one year old. I was invited to her first birthday party and almost overdid the celebrations. I was so overjoyed at the sight of the lovely baby-girl and above all, at the contentment of the parents who had dealt with an adult problem in an adult way.

From
Dr Jonathan Miles's
Casebook

Case 4

GLORIA

There are some cases the successful conclusion of which rouses very mixed feelings in a doctor. One is supremely happy to have been able to restore to health and happiness a human personality that it has been a pleasure to know; and with that goes a deep regret that, when the final consultation and examination are concluded, the last handshake exchanged, that patient will go away into the outside world from which he came, with the odds heavily against ever seeing him again. This is particularly so in specialists' practice generally, and very, very true in my own narrow field. The specialist in venereal diseases is not merely a doctor whom the average person does not want to consult; he is one – such is the attitude still prevalent to-day – with whom even a nodding acquaintance may set gossiping tongues a-wag.

I shall be very sorry to say godspeed and good-bye to Gloria. But, even more than with most of my cases, I am filled with delight and deep satisfaction that she was brought to me in time, and that I have been able to restore her to absolute normality with all the chances in a life whose existence was so tragically threatened. Failure in her case would have been a crime against humanity in the truest sense. It was, too, a case which shows, in a very striking way, how insidiously and subtly the curse of venereal disease may creep into an entirely innocent life and threaten it almost unnoticed. Because of these things it is Gloria's, out of all the hundreds of examples I might have chosen, which I have decided to introduce to you first.

Those who still harbour lurking doubts in their minds that venereal disease and active sin and immorality are indissolubly connected would do well to ponder deeply the bald facts of Gloria's case and ask themselves how their prejudices and misconceptions look in the light of those details. Gloria does not fit into any of the readymade classifications of moralists and generalizers. She is no 'good-time girl', as people call them for some reason quite beyond me, paying the price of folly. Nor is she one of the many who – in the cant phrase so full of righteous smugness – have yielded to temptation in a moment of weakness. Still less is she, or could she be, a representative of that pitiful class of women so often seen in VD clinics – wives suffering not for their own deeds but for the adventures of profligate or stupid husbands.

No, she belongs to none of these classes. For when Gloria was brought to me, a little over a year ago, she was barely fifteen years of age.

Of course, there are plenty of opportunities for girls of that age to contract venereal disease, as experience is continuing proving only too often. But no one, after five minutes' acquaintanceship with Gloria, could think for a moment that she was sexually precocious. As for the idea that she might be paying for the misconduct of her parents, no sane person could entertain the notion for a single instant. Her personal and her family records are alike blameless.

To some it may seem incredible – impossible, even – that Gloria should have had syphilis, the more terrible of the two principal venereal diseases. Yet it is a fact – a very important and striking fact, for it demonstrates in a most convincing way that the venereal diseases are not necessarily associated with sin or laxity or immorality – call it what you will – but can be contracted for precisely the same reasons or causes as one acquires other bacteria-borne diseases: a chance combination of circumstances that favour the transmission and rapid growth of the micro-organism.

Faced with an undoubted case of specific disease, the doctor's first and paramount responsibility is to ensure that every possible means is adopted for effecting a cure. It may be important, both for him and for the public health authorities, to know how, where, and when, the disease was contracted; in some instances – small-pox – for example – the resources of the State are employed for finding the answer to those questions. But such matters are, in the true sense, secondary; they should not be considered until the primary need for providing proper treatment has been satisfied and progress is being recorded.

I shall not, therefore, run ahead of my facts and seek to provide answers for the enigma of how, where, and when Gloria became infected with syphilis, but tell the story of this case as it presented itself to me, and I will add, at this stage, that at first Gloria's case was as much of a problem as regards its origins as it must be to those who have read so far.

It was on a day in March when she first came to me. The case was introduced to my department by a young doctor in general practice – a man whom I had met several times, and for whom a brilliant career was predicted if only because of his grim determination to take nothing for granted even to the extent of running the risk of being ridiculed for over-caution. To those qualities and his suspicious attitude, Gloria and her parents cannot fail to be everlastingly grateful. With no discredit to themselves, quite a number of medical men would certainly have overlooked the possibility of venereal disease, or, if it had crossed their minds, dismissed the idea as untenable in the light of the history of the case and the age of the patient.

Before Gloria came to the clinic, Dr Farman called on me. He was a trifle embarrassed and apologized for seeming to waste my time.

'Tell me about the case,' I said. 'You wouldn't be here unless you had suspicions, and my job is to sort out suspicions and hope to find that they're wrong.'

'If you find my suspicions wrong,' he answered, 'no one will be better pleased than me. You can laugh at me as much as you like for being over-cautious or even a bit mad.'

'I shan't laugh,' I commented. 'The greatest satisfaction one gets out of this job is being able to tell a patient that all his suspicions and fears are wrong – and that goes for doctors, too. But, of course, we don't do that unless we're satisfied first. Now go ahead.'

'I suppose VD is one of the last things I should think of,' he said, still a little on the defensive. 'But there it is. I shan't be satisfied till you rule it out – and I know that if you rule it out, I must be definitely wrong.'

'I'll do my very best to show that you are wrong,' I returned with a smile. 'Now, what about it? My time's valuable, if yours isn't.'

He relaxed at this sally. 'The patient is a girl of fifteen,' he explained. 'The family – her father and mother and herself – are regular patients of mine, amongst my oldest – not that they worry me much. They're all of them decent, healthy people who're very rarely ill. I hadn't seen any of them for nine months before the mother brought Gloria to me. The family history strikes me as important and it makes my suspicions appear all the more ridiculous.'

'Family history is vitally important, as you know, in these cases,' I observed. 'There's no history of VD, and you've never had any sort of suspicions of it in the family?'

He shook his head. 'No – quite definitely. I've overhauled all three of them from time to time, and apart from the physical indications – or lack of them – they're all remarkably frank. Ideal patients in fact.'

'Go on,' I nodded.

'Gloria was sent to me for general malaise,' he continued. 'Nothing definitely wrong. She complained of headaches and general lassitude. Her digestion had started to go wrong. Occasionally, for no overt reason, she'd run a temperature. Well, a girl of that age does sometimes start to behave erratically, as you know – especially when she shows signs of anaemia, as Gloria did. That was what struck me at once. She'd suddenly become quite noticeably anaemic, and I'd never seen anything of that sort in her before, though, naturally, when one has a girl of that age under examination, it's something one bears strongly in mind.'

'You gave her general tonic treatment, I suppose?' I suggested.

He nodded. 'Yes. It was the obvious thing to do and I suppose I should have left it at that and hoped for the best – that she'd grow out of it. But I don't like doing that sort of thing. If something is wrong, there must be a reason, and I like to find it out. Besides, the deterioration in Gloria's condition was relatively sudden. Nothing in her history, as I knew it, and I thought I knew it pretty well, suggested the course events had taken.'

'I admit,' I said, 'that syphilis could and does produce these symptoms in certain atypical cases during the secondary stage. But frankly I don't see that even a man with a suspicious mind like yours could jump to that diagnosis merely on what you've told me so far. A dozen or more conditions might account for this picture.'

Again he nodded. 'I know. But that isn't quite all. I'm going through the case stage by stage. I gave her general treatment, as you suggested, but she didn't respond at all satisfactorily – in fact, the general malaise tended to get worse. I don't say she was under continuous treatment all this time. After the first interview, in fact, I did not see her again for some time, and it was at this second consultation that her mother looked really anxious.

'Rather understandably, she was taking a poor view of things. The girl was getting more and more depressed because she was unable to carry out her usual mode of life. Gloria's a budding musician, you know, and I should say she had something more than average talent and promise, though I'm not suggesting she'll ever make an international celebrity – which may be just as well for her. Here her principal complaint arose. She found she couldn't concentrate on her practice and studies any longer and that was a very serious thing for her indeed. It's really all she ever cares about. Every spare minute she has she spends at the piano or studying books on music. That naturally depressed her and a vicious circle was set up in the usual way.'

'Yes. But we're still getting no nearer to what caused you to suspect VD,' I interposed, glancing – I hope not too, ostentatiously – at my watch.

'Oh, yes, we are,' he responded, with a bright grin. 'I can see you are beginning to get impatient. It was at the second consultation and examination that I began to be puzzled. I tried a mild psychological investigation but it proved more or less negative, and in the course of that, one or two things that later seemed significant came out. I asked Gloria and her mother precisely what depressed her. The mother replied that everything did, including the most absurd trifles. For example, she said, she'd found Gloria in tears because she kept finding hairs on her brush and comb, and she was frightened she was going bald.'

'Ah!' I breathed.

He smiled slightly but made no comment on my suddenly rising interest.

'The long and the short of it is,' he resumed, 'that I overhauled her again, but the results were practically the same – nothing very suggestive, though I did detect a very slight rash, rather scattered in its distribution. She couldn't account for it, and it was so slight she'd barely noticed it herself.

'Well, there it is,' he went on. 'It's not a very convincing case. But I've turned it over and over in my mind, and the possibility – the outside possibility – of syphilis is the only thing I can entertain. There's the rash, to which otherwise I can't give a name convincingly. There's that little chance scrap of information about the falling hair – girls of her age don't shed their hair like that. Well, there's not much more I can say about it. I've had to put aside all questions of causation. The girl's *virgo intacta*, by the way, and no questions I've put to her throw any light on it. All the same, I think she ought to be examined and have a proper test.'

'Yes,' I returned. 'There's no harm in it anyway. It's not a very typical case – but then what case of syphilis is? The textbooks give you a description of what they call the "normal form", but how often do you see it in practice? Very rarely. You're a brave man, by the way, to follow it up like that. What did the parents say to your suggestion?'

'They were just too staggered to speak to begin with, but I pointed out to them that I recommended a specialist's examination merely as a wise precaution. There was a suspicion in my mind that it might be VD so it was proper to have that set at rest before we looked for anything else.'

'No sense of outrage?' I asked. 'No angry attempts to protect the virtue of their daughter against the foul suggestion?' I was anxious to find out what sort of people I had to deal with so that I might take the right approach to them.

'No. They're a sensible crowd,' he replied, 'and they take the view that our old friend the spirochaete is no more an agent of the Devil himself than any other disease bacterium. They're incredulous, of course. I can't say how she got it or even make a guess, if it is that. They have no idea either. I think they rather look on it all as a wild goose chase, and briefly I hope they're right. I've never wanted to be proved wrong so much before.'

'I'll do my best to satisfy your wishes,' I said rising. 'And they'll be here at two o'clock to-morrow afternoon? That's the arrangement, I think.'

He nodded. 'Yes. And thanks a lot.'

The interview had taken a long time, and there was no opportunity to think it over till the evening came. And then, passing the case in review, I could not help feeling that Dr Farman was being rather over-cautious. If I had not known him pretty well, both personally and by reputation, I might easily have suspected him of being one of those young men who take a delight in ignoring the obvious and go chasing after the wildest possible hypothesis, merely to show how very clever and knowledgeable they are. But such a course did not fit in at all with what I knew of Farman. As he had presented it to me, the case looked unconvincing; he had more than admitted that it was of the slenderest kind. But I knew very well that it is not always possible to put down in black and white or express in words everything on which a doctor bases his diagnosis and suspicions. There are small, almost imperceptible, signs that are highly suggestive to the eye of experience yet elusive of expression or description. In their work in this so-called scientific age, doctors are not supposed to take actions on what are popularly known as 'hunches' or intuitions; yet, in fact, it is precisely such indefinable things which often lead a doctor in his investigations and which prove, in the long run, the most reliable. And why should it not be so? Is it not the development of the power of intuitive judgment alongside scientific analysis which gives the experienced doctor his superiority over the inexperienced? Is not experience, in fact, but the development of a special sense and power of association?

The next day, Gloria and her mother came to see me at the appointed hour. I took an instant liking to both of them. They were clearly very worried and the mother was quite unable to understand why the consultation was necessary. But her doctor, a man in whom she trusted, had advised it and she accepted his guidance in the proper spirit. Since that was her attitude, I made my examination at once, before entering into explanation and possible argument, which might lead anywhere. It was not a very convincing examination. There was certainly the rash in which Farman had referred, but it was very slight, and its discovery was a credit to his thoroughness, for it could be seen only under certain conditions of lighting and even then did not show up very well.

It was this which I made my chief point in stressing the need for a proper blood test and laboratory investigation of the girl's condition. Having gone so far, they must, I said, take the thing to its proper conclusion. I myself, I explained, could not say 'yes' or 'no', or even entertain any opinion at all, until I had had such tests made, and I felt sure that they would be storing up trouble for themselves, in the form of constantly recurring doubts whenever the girl was ill, if they decided now not to allow me to complete my work.

'Look on it as a proper precaution, like having the brakes of a car tested,' I said to the mother. 'If they're all right, so much the better. You'll feel happier and safer because you know they're all right.'

'Very well, doctor,' she replied in a low voice. 'If you think it necessary, it must be done. I leave everything entirely to you.' She shook her head wearily. 'But I don't understand it at all. It seems impossible to me – utterly impossible. Surely you can get this horrible thing in only one way?'

'Unfortunately that general belief leads to a great deal of trouble,' I said grimly. 'There are several possible ways of contracting the venereal diseases without sexual intercourse in the ordinary sense. But while people believe that they have to have intercourse to run the risk of infection, and while some official propaganda, excellent in other ways, seems to confirm that belief, we shan't get all the way to conquering this disease. I hope Gloria is free from the disease. If not, have no doubt that we can cure her quite rapidly. And don't get ideas about moral tar-brushes.'

'Very well,' she said again, in the same low, resigned voice. 'I hope you are all wrong, doctor, about Gloria, but if you're not, you must promise to help me to get to the bottom of this business.'

I promised her – not merely to pacify her, but also because I, too, was filled with an overwhelming desire to find out the facts of as strange a case as any I had handled. So I made arrangements for Gloria to come the next day when I should be ready to take the blood and other samples necessary for the laboratory tests.

These examinations include a microscopical inspection of the blood and other fluids and several specific tests beside the well-known Wassermann test. By means of these tests, the existence of the Spirochaeta pallida, the micro-organism causing syphilis, can be determined and an estimate of the extent of the infection made.

The Wassermann test – being the first in the field – has often been written of as though it were a magic touchstone, but though it is an essential and perhaps the most important weapon in the doctor's armoury for detecting syphilis, it is rather oracular in its messages. For example, though a positive test does establish beyond reasonable doubt that the patient under examination has contracted the disease there are certain conditions of the blood that may give a positive reaction though there is no syphilis; luckily these are rare and they can be recognised fairly easily by other means. Sometime the test gives an ambiguous answer on which it is impossible to decide one way or the other. Again, if the test is negative, it does not by any means clear the patient of suspicion, for if the test is repeated a week, one month, or even several months later, the reaction may be strongly positive.

Whenever there is the slightest doubt, therefore, the only course is to test again and again and to employ other, more sensitive tests; it is only when a series of tests repeated several times over a period of months have been constantly negative that one can allow oneself to relax one's suspicions. Diagnosing syphilis does not depend however, on one or more tests, nor merely on the laboratory investigations as a whole; it is the complete picture that must be studied.

For these reasons, it is equally impossible to say at once with certainty that any case has been cured. The signs and symptoms may have disappeared – as they do fairly quickly with modern methods of treatment – the tests may be unquestionably negative, but it is only when such tests have been repeated at intervals over a period of a year or more that the doctor is prepared to discharge the case – and even then he has to impress on the patient the vital necessity of consulting him again should there be the slightest cause to suspect a reappearance. The spirochaete is not only one of the most malignant enemies of man, it is also one of the most persistent and insidious, carrying out, as it were, its terrible work in dark streets.

I did not expect any difficulties in diagnosis in Gloria's case. If she had contracted syphilis – though how she might have done so was a problem in itself – the presence of the spirochaete should be fairly easy to show. For it is one of the most curious things about this extraordinary disease that, in the initial stages, when the external signs are often of the grossest kind, the micro-organism is frequently elusive and the first tests are negative. On the other hand, in the early generalized secondary stage, when, as in Gloria's case, the signs and symptoms add up to a little more than a suspicion, the tests are more often than not markedly positive. So if it were in truth secondary syphilis that was Gloria's trouble, I felt that our doubts and fears would soon be set at rest one way or the other.

Unfortunately, the results were only too satisfactory from the scientific point of view. There could be no doubt that Gloria was suffering from a widespread general syphilitic infection. When the young doctor called on me to learn the finding, his comment summed up precisely my own feelings.

'My God!' he exclaimed when he had studied the laboratory reports. 'No doubt about that. If ever there was a case in which I longed to be proved wrong, this is it, and it doesn't give me the slightest thrill to be proved right.'

Naturally, Gloria's mother was distraught when she heard the news, but she faced the situation bravely.

'You can cure it, doctor, can't you?' she asked almost pleadingly. 'I mean, it's a real cure, and she won't go about with this horrible thing hanging over her head all her life.'

'Yes,' I replied. 'We can cure it, though it may take a little time, of course. You were lucky in your choice of doctor, by the way. Thanks to his suspicions, we're taking this in reasonably good time. Later on we should still have been able to cure, but the disease might possibly have made marks that could never have been completely eradicated.'

She was silent for a little while as though reflecting on this sombre thought. Then she looked up at me inquiringly.

'I suppose you use penicillin nowadays,' she remarked. 'It seems wonderful stuff.'

I nodded slowly. 'Yes, penicillin is proving a great help to us in cases like this, and Gloria, will be treated with it. But I'm sure you agree with me that we must make assurance doubly sure.'

'Yes,' she said intently. 'You must do everything – please.'

'Of course, we shall,' I answered. 'That's why I shall give Gloria a combined treatment. Together with the penicillin, she shall have an intensive course of arsenic preparations.'

'Arsenic?' she echoed in surprise. 'I didn't know you used that.'

'It was the standard treatment until we had penicillin and the other antibiotic drugs,' I returned. 'You have heard of the famous '606' – salvarsan?'

'Yes, as a matter of fact I saw that film, *The Magic Bullet*,' she replied. (This film told the story of Dr Ehrlich and his introduction of salvarsan for the treatment of syphilis.)

'That's known as arsphenamine – an organic compound of arsenic,' I explained. 'You see, cases treated with penicillin, or with some of the other antiobiotics, do respond very rapidly, and the results are almost invariably highly satisfactory. In Gloria's case I propose to use penicillin, or if she happens to be allergic to it, some other antibiotic drug to clear up the signs as quickly and as easily as possible and to make quite sure of the end result, I will also use arseno-therapy.'

She nodded. 'I'm not sure that I fully understand it all,' she said, 'but I'm confident you'll do everything you can – everything. I would much rather die myself than that Gloria should go through life with – that.'

'Set your mind at rest,' I insisted. 'We'll get the treatment going, and then we'll set about trying to find out how it happened.'

'Yes,' she said emphatically. 'We must do that.'

For myself, I am quite satisfied that the penicillin treatment by itself is normally sufficient, so is the treatment with the other antibiotic drugs, though, as with all drugs, there are some cases that do not respond to it and there is a small proportion of relapses after apparent cure. Full treatment with the older arsenical drugs, of which 606 was the pioneer (though it had been largely superseded by improved forms) used to occupy as much as a year or longer. Later, good results were obtained with more intensive methods of treatment of several weeks' duration only – though here again insufficient experience had then been collected to say what the final results of these treatments would be as regards a lasting cure. Injections with penicillin effect an immense reduction in time. Normally a week or a little more suffices for a full course of treatment, doses of the drug being introduced into the muscle at intervals of three to six hours for a period of seven or eight days.

The speed of the method does not, of course, in any way lessen the need for subsequent surveillance of the patient; in fact, our incomplete knowledge at the present time makes regular inspection and laboratory checks rather more necessary.

In Gloria's case I decided to administer the maximum dosage of penicillin over seven and a half days, during which time she would also have a couple of injections of neoarsphenamine – one of the successors of '606' – and one of bismuth. This would be followed during the ensuing nine weeks by a course of neoarsphenamine and bismuth injections. By these means I hoped not only to dispel the disease but also to provide a complete protection against the tragedy of its recurrence.

There is no need to go into the details of the progress of the case. She responded to treatment remarkably well, and several times I felt that I was ridiculously over-cautious in submitting her to the comparative rigours of the arseno-therapy. The penicillin, which she tolerated very well, had cleared away every sign and symptom, and the Wassermann tests were unambiguously and continuously negative – so were also all other tests. A fortnight after the penicillin course had been completed, we made the usual routine test for infection of the cerebro-spinal fluid, which is withdrawn by the well-known procedure of lumbar puncture. Invasion of this fluid by the spirochaete can have the most serious and lasting consequences. The tests were all negative.

When the combined treatment had been finally concluded, Gloria was put on the surveillance list. She came to me monthly for a thorough examination, during which blood and other samples were taken for test. Not once during the whole of the time she had been under control have there been the slightest signs of relapse or reinfection. In my mind, I am convinced that she is completely cured and that she is free to enjoy to the full the happy life to which she is surely entitled.

It was while I had her under treatment that I was able to talk to her and win her confidence in the most complete degree. I flatter myself that she came to look on me not merely as her doctor but also as a very good friend – which I hope I always shall be to her. And as a result of this happy relationship, which means so much between doctor and patient and contributes always to unchecked progress, I was able, at long last, to uncover the mystery of how she became infected.

Her favourite topic was her music. Sooner or later her talk always came round to that, and it was clear that it was her overriding passion in life. Nothing pleased her more than that I was able to provide her with a good radiogram and a supply of pianoforte records, which could not be played often enough for her during the time she necessarily spent in the clinic. Her conversation showed plainly that she had little interest in the things that occupy most girls of her age. In particular, she had a marked distaste for parties, and spoke with especial disfavour of one that she had attended during the Christmas season before she had come to me.

I asked her why it had been so unpleasant for her.

'There was a horrible man there,' she replied, grimacing at the mere memory. 'They called him Uncle Jack – I don't know his real name. I hated him the first time I saw him. But he made a dead set at me, and I wanted to run away and hide, but I didn't want to spoil Betty's party by being silly. We had a few dances and every time he came and asked me to dance with him. And when we played those stupid kissing games he always contrived to get hold of me. He's ghastly.' She shuddered.

I pricked up my ears. There was nothing at all tangible on which I could base the slanderous thought running through my mind that this Uncle Jack – obviously the unpleasant kind that likes pawing young girls – might be the cause of her infection. But it was the only glimpse of an explanation – unlikely enough, it was true – that I had had; and I resolved to follow it up. I said nothing to Gloria, of course, but I made a careful note of the facts, and a little judicious questioning, drew out a few more pieces of information about the man. It was as I suspected: he appeared a wholly undesirable person, certainly not the kind that should be invited to a party of young people.

Next day I mentioned, in confidence, my vague suspicions to her mother.

'Well, of course, I can't say,' she replied. 'All I can say is that I was very much annoyed when I heard that he'd been at Betty's party. He's the last person on earth I should have wanted Gloria to meet, and I can't understand what Betty's mother was about inviting him. Everyone talks about him, and though I'm no gossip, I do think there's no smoke without fire.'

Rather reluctantly she gave me, under pressure, the man's name and address, which she happened to know.

So far, so good, I thought. But the next step was not so easy. I could not present myself at 'Uncle Jack's' house and confront him with a blunt accusation of being a suspected syphilitic. If I did so, I should lay myself open to legal consequences, to say nothing of the probability of more immediate and violent action. It seemed an insoluble problem with the law at it stood. Even if I trumped up a case – as I wildly thought of doing at one time – and reported him to the local Medical Officer of Health as having been named by two patients in the clinic as the source of their infection, he could still hold out; and I might easily end my career with ignominy. That course was obviously impossible.

I do not know how I should have got to the bottom of the affair had not luck helped me in a remarkable way. For the purposes of a scientific paper I was preparing to read before a medical society, I happened to be going through recent records – and there I found the name of 'Uncle Jack'. I could barely believe my eyes. It seemed almost incredible. But there it was, and there could be no doubt that there was no confusion of identities. Name and address were identical.

His case was of a familiar – a too unpleasantly familiar – type. He had come to the clinic, under pressure from his own doctor, in November of the previous year, and his infection had been established at once. He had proved a recalcitrant patient, resisting all advice; and, after a little while, as so often happens with people of his anti-social and irresponsible type, he had simply discontinued his visits for treatment. We could not compel him to continue; the law does not provide for that. He was one more of those moral criminals who, knowing they are infected, are prepared to go about spreading the disease.

I studied the history of his case. By about January, I estimated, the disease would have become fairly generalized and there would have been some degree of infection of the mouth. In such a state, it was possible he might have conveyed the disease by kissing. Everything fitted in.

In the light of these suggestive findings, I questioned Gloria anew. Had she at any time experienced any special discomfort of the mouth or tongue – in particular had she noticed any spot or sore in those regions?

She seemed surprised but she cudgelled her brains in her efforts to remember. In the end, she told me she had noticed no sore or spot in her mouth after the party, but the 'old one had still been there'.

'The old one?' I repeated. 'What was that?'

'I'd had it about a week,' she replied. 'I stuck a fork into my tongue and it was quite a nasty place. Mummy joked about it and said I wouldn't be able to eat anything at Betty's party. It lasted a long time.'

That was enough for me. The spirochaeta pallida finds its way into the body more readily through the mucous membranes than through the skin, and it is only likely to take a firm hold when there is some break in the surface – a small scratch is sufficient. Yet here was a girl with what she described as a 'nasty place', unhealed, on the tongue, engaging in kissing games with an uncured syphilitic, probably in a state of oral infection. I felt that the search was over, and the mystery explained.

Now I took my courage in both hands. I called on 'Uncle Jack'. I told him that I had come to make a last appeal to him to resume treatment or at any rate to have another examination. He laughed at me, but in the end, when I had painted a very vivid picture of his own last probable state and of the danger he was causing to others, he submitted. His infection was still very active. More than that, he had marked areas of diseased tissue in the mouth and lip areas. My case was as complete as I was ever likely to make it.

For myself, I do not doubt that that innocent kissing game was the cause of Gloria's infection. Nothing else I have found could explain it even remotely. But of course the type of proof that would satisfy either a scientist or a court of law cannot be brought forward. It is, logically, nothing more than a probability – yet it is, to my mind, so high a probability as to be almost a certainty.

To some it may seem surprising, if my guesses are right, that Gloria did not notice anything wrong with her mouth, but this is not at all unusual. The primary chancre – the sore – which is usually the first outward sign of syphilis is frequently so small as to remain unnoticed even when it is on a part of the body that is easily inspected. In the mouth, it often passes unsuspected since little or no pain accompanies it as a rule.

And in Gloria's case there was a double reason for its remaining undetected, for she had already had a sore on her tongue and would ascribe any discomfort or visible mark to that cause. All her initial troubles were connected with the mouth and throat, moreover, which adds weight to my conjectures.

That, then, is the case of Gloria, happy in its final outcome (as nearly all cases are if handled properly) yet tragic in its main and compelling features. For me it had great clinical interest, though the actual progress and treatment of the disease were unremarkable in the text-book sense. But it has a greater and deeper significance than its medical details provide, for it does reveal, in the most striking way, how syphilis can come in the most innocent guise and is likely to remain unrecognized except by the most searching eyes, such as those of Gloria's doctor.

Of these general aspects, I shall have more – much more – to say later. Let us take the case of Gloria as it stands and think over it. In itself, it provides overwhelming evidence of the need for completely revising many of the most strongly held popular misconceptions about venereal diseases in general and syphilis in particular.

CHRISTOPHER

Christopher is a brave and realistic man. And because he has those qualities he is enjoying today a happiness that might otherwise have been wrecked. He showed, when he consulted me, what I believe to be one of the highest forms of moral courage; he came to admit that he had played the fool and was ready to pay the price, if necessary, of his folly. That is why he is today again a healthy man – and the two persons who mean most to him in life have been saved from a major disaster.

To me, Christopher's case had an all too familiar appearance. As he explained the details to me, I could have closed my eyes and imagined that I was hearing once more the pitiful, stumbling story of a hundred patients who had preceded him. Something like it is recorded in practically every one of the books that have been written about venereal disease, but that does not make its message any the less telling. It sounds a warning that cannot be too often repeated, teaches a lesson that must be hammered home ceaselessly.

Some people seem to think that the only patients dealt with at VD clinics are the sweepings of the moral gutters. They believe that those who have contracted this terrible disease are marked out, like lepers, from the rest of mankind. The tragedy is that this attitude is due not to ignorance (unless it be wilful, for the facts are easy enough to come by these days) but to prejudice. The case of Christopher is typical of thousands and completely gives the lie to that stupid, dangerous misconception. There was nothing of the moral degenerate, the roué, or the profligate, about him; he was a perfect example of the average, decent-living citizen, and no one looking at or knowing him could form any other conclusion.

He was not yet thirty, and, with his qualities of steadiness and integrity, he was bound to go far in the service of the insurance company with which he was associated. During the war, he had a most distinguished record, for he was awarded the Military Cross, was twice mentioned in dispatches, and finished with the rank of a major in the Airborne Division with which he served. Just before the war ended, he had married a charming girl whom he had met as a nurse in the military hospital to which he was sent to convalesce after being wounded in Normandy.

Life seemed good and hopeful to Christopher and his wife when they settled down to peacetime conditions. He had a good job and the determination to get on. They were among the very fortunate ones who had succeeded in finding a small house of their own, and Christopher's salary was sufficient to enable him to run a small car. The Lady Fortune seemed to have made him her friend in peace as well as in war.

He led a quiet, uneventful life, happy in his home, and there seemed no reason why it should not be continued. But Fate plays curious tricks, and her special delight is to strike down those who appear to have found the secret of contentment.

It happened like this. Diana, his wife, had gone away to spend a few days with her parents, who lived in the country, and he was to join them at the week-end and bring Diana back with him in the car on the Sunday night. She left home on the Tuesday, and on Wednesday an evil chance threw Eddy across his path.

Eddy had been a brother officer during the war. He was one of those men to whom war seems the natural state of affairs and who find peace dull and unexciting. He had never been one of Christopher's intimates, for Eddy's way of life in all things was hectic and risky, and Christopher, even when he was a soldier, preferred the safer and less eventful paths. There was very little in common between them.

They had met in a London street. Christopher had bestowed a passing, and not wholly approving, glance on the man who jostled him on the pavement. He did not like suits, however well cut, that had grossly over-built shoulders; nor did he take kindly to men who wore carnation buttonholes in mid-December. There was something flashy and repulsive about such details in Christopher's eyes.

The stranger turned with a word of apology, for he had stumbled quite heavily against Christopher, and as he did so his eyes opened wide in surprise and a delight that may or may not have been feigned.

'Why, if it isn't old Christopher!' he exclaimed. 'Of all the luck! I haven't seen you since we were together at Hereford, old boy. Where the hell have you been hiding yourself?'

Christopher smiled. 'Oh, I've been pushing around, you know. Not much time for looking up the old gang. You see, I'm taking an exam soon, so naturally I don't get about.'

'What's the game?' asked Eddy, producing a long, flat gold cigarette case and proffering it to Christopher.

'Insurance,' replied Christopher. 'I'm hoping to get into the actuarial side.'

Eddy made a face. 'You're welcome to it all,' he said. 'You always were the brainy type, but it doesn't mean a thing to me. I've got a little show of my own – doing fine. These days you can sell anything to anybody, and I'm sitting pretty. How are you fixed, old man? Come and have lunch with me?'

Christopher shook his head. 'Thanks a lot,' he replied. 'I'm due back at the office in twenty minutes, and I've got stacks of stuff to get through.'

'And I don't suppose you get as much for it as I make in a little deal over a drink,' commented Eddy. 'Takes all sorts to make a world, I suppose. But, look here, meet me this evening and we'll go places together.'

Christopher hesitated. He had no particular wish to 'go places' with Eddy, for Eddy in his peacetime guise was even less attractive to him than Eddy the soldier had been. But he felt lost and lonely without Diana; the thought of going back to an empty house had been returning to him at intervals throughout the day, each time with a greater chilliness. He was in the mood to be tempted, and his reluctance did not last long.

'OK,' he replied. 'I'd love to. Where shall we meet?'

'Know Merci's?' asked Eddy.

Christopher shook his head. His knowledge of West End bars was limited.

Eddy told him where it was. 'I'll be there about six,' he said, 'and we'll knock back a couple and then go and have a spot of dinner. If I'm not there, tell Hugo the barman you're a friend of mine, and he'll see you get what you want. OK, then. Six o'clock. I'll be seeing you.'

He waved extravagantly and strolled on, leaving Christopher half inclined to chase after him and cancel the arrangement. But he did not, though every passing hour of the afternoon increased his regrets that he had yielded to Eddy's pressure.

With some difficulty Christopher found Merci's, a small, expensive, and rather dubious bar in one of the mysterious streets behind Regent Street. It was nearly half past six when he pushed open the orange, black and red door, to be met by a clamour of voices and a wave of stuffy, smoke-laden air. There was no sign of Eddy, but he filtered through the crush and eventually caught sight of him sitting on a high stool in the corner at the far end of the long bar, which flanked the entire right-hand wall.

Eddy nodded easily at him.

'Hullo, old man. Almost given you up,' he said. 'Got held up?'

'No,' replied Christopher slipping on the stool that, by some miracle, Eddy had contrived to reserve for him. 'Just couldn't find the place.'

'You should've taken a taxi, old boy. Always the best way when you're not sure of your objective. Every taximan knows this dive.'

Christopher said nothing. Taxis were not of his world.

'What'll you have, old man?' asked Eddy.

'Oh, I don't mind,' replied Christopher uncomfortably, feeling thoroughly out of his element. 'Lager.'

Eddy raised his eyebrows. 'Really? Plenty of spirits, you know, here. You don't know what shortages mean, do you, Hugo?' he added as an aside to the barman. 'I always think beer spoils your palate for dinner, but have it your own way.'

'All right, then,' said Christopher miserably. 'I'll have a Scotch.' He looked about him. He did not like the men; they were all of Eddy's type. Still less did he like the women. There were too many fur capes, to many diamonds, too much emphatic make-up, for his liking. Yet, under the influence of two or three double whiskies, he began to enjoy it in spite of himself. It was a new experience.

By the time Eddy decided it was time for dinner, Christopher was feeling a trifle fuddled, probably less to the effect of the drinks than of the stagnant noisy atmosphere. Eddy smiled at him and, placing his hand under Christopher's arm, led him round the corner to a large, over-magnificent American car, scintillating with chromium fittings.

'Lovely job,' remarked Eddy. 'One of my little deals, you know. Managed to get hold of it – well, it doesn't matter how. Already had offers of twice what I gave for it, but I'm holding out till they cough up what I want. I'll get it.'

'You like large profits,' said Christopher.

'Who doesn't,' returned Eddy, with a shrug. 'And the beauty of it is that they can't dock you for income-tax on things like this. It's the only worth-while racket these days.'

He took Christopher to a small restaurant where he was greeted as though he owned the place. The manager and the head waiter hovered round the table and proposed, between them, a menu that suggested price was no object and also that inflation meant very little as far as Eddy was concerned. It was extravagant dining in its true meaning. And in addition to the rich food, there was plenty of drink of most expensive foreign vintage. Christopher, no expert in wines, does not remember what he had, though he vaguely recalls a particularly vicious cocktail, wine bottles of two different kinds, and brandy served in a huge balloon glass.

It was late when they left the restaurant, and Christopher's mind was now far from clear. He blinked at his watch. To his dismay he saw that it was almost eleven o'clock.

'I say, Eddy,' he said in agitation. 'I shall have to shift. My last train goes at eleven twenty-five.'

'Don't worry about that, old boy,' remarked Eddy. 'We may as well make a night of it. I'll look after you. We're just getting warmed up. Grand show.'

'But ...' protested Christopher weakly. He confessed that he

wanted nothing more than to be among the familiar things of
his own home again. He thought of the cat, which should have
been fed hours ago, and he experienced a flush of guilt.

'Come on, old man,' insisted Eddy, piloting him into the
car. 'You told me the missis was away, so what the hell have
you got to worry about?'

From that moment, Christopher's memory for details fails
him. He was taken to a night-club called, he believes, The
Tattered Bathrobe, though he cannot swear to it. He is sure
about the word 'tattered' in the title because he recalls that it
struck him as so very apt. This was Merci's in an even more
intense way. Drink of all kind flowed freely. There was a band
to add to the general hubbub, and a small dance floor where
couples stood stock still, locked in each other's arms. In short
it was typical of the night club of the twenties and the bottle
party of today – a place to which people go for the 'pleasure' of
drinking, picking up partners of the opposite sex, and making
a noise to hide their utter emptiness and boredom.

He was quite drunk now, and it is difficult to sort out from
his memories what is fact and what due to hallucination
induced by excessive alcohol. But he has no doubt of one thing
that happened. He recalls with complete clarity that when
Eddy had conducted him downstairs and out into the fresh
air, which was like a breath from Heaven to him, they were
accompanied by two women; and he is quite certain that those
women, painted and peroxided, were nothing more than
common prostitutes, despite their expensive clothes and lovely
furs. One went in the front with Eddy. The other came in the
back of the car with him. After that his recollections dim a
little, but he has vague impressions of being in a flat
somewhere, of more drinks, and of the woman putting her
arms about him and leading him across the hall to a small
bedroom.

When he awoke next morning, it was broad daylight. He
looked round him with a start, for the room was quite
unfamiliar. His watch told him it was nearly half past eleven.
The thought of the office caused him to attempt to rise from
the bed. He fell back. His head was splitting, his whole body
ached. He felt as though he would rather be dead.

Then Eddy came in – suave, calm, smiling, and clad in a gorgeous silk dressing-gown.

'How d'you feel, old boy?' he asked lightly. 'It was a whale of a night wasn't it? And you sure know how to pick 'em. I could have done with a spot of that blonde myself.' He handed Christopher a glass he was carrying; it had an effervescing fluid in it. 'Better drink this, old man. I don't know what it is, but my chemist makes it up for hangovers, and it's just marvellous.'

Christopher drank. His mouth was parched and dry, and the drink was cool and refreshing.

'But the office, Eddy!' he gasped miserably. 'The office ...'

'Don't worry, old boy,' returned Eddy, grinning. 'I rang them up for you an hour ago and said you were ill and wouldn't be in today. That's OK. Think of everything, don't I?'

'Thanks,' said Christopher weakly, feeling more ashamed than ever. He slipped back into the bedclothes.

'Yes, you'd better lie up for a little while,' said Eddy. 'I've got a date for lunch, so you stay there till I come back. Then we'll fix you up.'

It was late afternoon when Christopher, feeling better now, dressed and prepared to depart. He declined Eddy's offer to motor him home; he preferred to arrive in the usual way, as though he was returning from the office.

'Oh, by the way, Eddy,' he said, feeling in his pocket for his wallet, 'how much do I owe you?'

Eddy chuckled and made a large gesture. 'Forget it, old boy. Show was on me last night.'

'But really, I must stand my corner – really I must.' Christopher opened the wallet and his eyes grew round. 'But what's happened?' he exclaimed. 'I had nearly thirty quid in there and it's all gone! Have I been robbed or what?'

Eddy sighed a little patronizingly. 'My dear, Christopher,' he said, 'surely you don't think you can have a hell of a time with a swell dame like that blonde for nothing, do you? After all, the girl's got to live, you know. You can't have it all ways.'

'No,' said Christopher dully. 'No.'

In the train going home, he was overcome by shame and

remorse. Eddy's last remark had stung him.

'All the best, old man,' he said. 'Good job the little woman's away, isn't it? We all need a break sometime, you know.'

He had wanted to punch Eddy's smiling face, but he held himself in; that would not put things straight. It had been a relief to say goodbye at the station.

It was just the story of a plain debauch that must happen dozens of times every week, especially when a man meets an old comrade and they decide to make a night of it together. It starts off innocently enough but how often does it end as Christopher's escapade did? Not always perhaps on the lavish scale of Eddy's outing, but the principle is the same. For whether the scene be a questionable expensive party or a dingy room off the Charing Cross Road, the drunken men who have celebrated take their dreary pleasure in a way to which no animal would descend. So, in a moment of stupor, they lay the foundations of a life-time's trouble.

To a man like Christopher, the mental remorse and self-accusation which follow events of this kind are more than a sufficient payment for the doubtful enjoyment they afford. In the next couple of days, Christopher underwent the torments of utter self-abasement. Every item in the lonely house seemed to accuse him silently, and he dreaded the meeting with Diana. Many times he felt that he ought to confess everything to her, but at last he decided it was better to let sleeping dogs lie; and when, on the Saturday afternoon, he arrived for the week-end at his father-in-law's house, he believed that he had succeeded in relegating the affair to the status of a skeleton in a cupboard that must be kept tightly locked. Once or twice he thought Diana looked at him rather curiously and intently as though she found something odd in his manner or appearance, but that may have been due to his guilty conscience. By the end of the following week, he was able to go about his business troubled by nothing more than a sudden memory, which, however, still had the power to stab sharply and wound deeply.

But three weeks later, the whole unhappy affair descended on him again like a black and evil cloud, and he found himself staring tragedy in the face. Superficially there was nothing to justify it, and that is why I have described him as a man of moral courage. Diana told him she was going to have a baby. He was pleased beyond measure – for the moment. And then the full implications dawned on him.

Christopher was no ignoramus. He had learnt a good deal about venereal diseases while he had been in the Army, and he had seen more than sufficient of the havoc they can cause. It was because of this that he woke in the night overcome with panic. Suppose ... suppose that girl – he barely remembered what she looked like – suppose she hadn't been 'clean', as he put it? There was Diana, Diana who was perfectly innocent and trusting. More than Diana there was the child. The possibilities nearly drove him mad.

Try as he could, it was impossible to drive away the haunting thoughts. He tried to tell himself that girls like that would certainly look after themselves. He had not picked her up in the streets; she moved in well-to-do circles ... But he knew that was mere self-delusion. Disease is no respecter of class or wealth or anything else. One finds it at least as much among the rich as among the poor. It strikes the virtuous no less than the wicked. The girl led a life which exposed her to infection, and she might harbour it quite unknowingly. Almost certainly, being what she was, she would not consciously hand it on, but he knew that it was difficult to detect the disease in anyone, and particularly difficult in a woman.

All the next day and the day after, he was tormented by the thoughts. He examined his body carefully, looking for some tell-tale sign. There was none. But this again, being a well-informed young man, he knew was no certain guide. It was at this stage that he took the highly sensible decision to consult me. In a properly instructed and well-organized world, taking such a step would be regarded as no more than common prudence in the circumstances – like seeing a doctor about a persistent sore throat. But in the world we live in, it is only those of high moral courage who take it. As a rule, men and women wait until there are overt signs before they rush in a panic to the nearest VD clinic – and even then, the majority postpone the dreaded visit for as long as possible, doing everything they can to explain away (and sometimes charm away) the suspicious sore or chancre. In the majority of cases, I think I can say, patients who come to VD clinics have tried to drive away the chancre – the first sign of the disease – by the use of antiseptics and ointments and the like. By so doing they increase the already great difficulties of diagnosis and frequently lull themselves into a sense of false security.

He told me his story haltingly at first, hesitating and gabbling his words by turns. But when he found that no moral judgments were passed on him and that my attitude was perfectly friendly and matter-of-fact, he grew more confident and recalled, one by one, all the details I have already given. Doctors in VD clinics share with psychiatrists the need for at least one characteristic: they must acquire the art of ignoring or smoothing away their patients' moral difficulties and obstacles, and they must be ready for the probability of mis-statements arising out of those difficulties. Nor must they show any condemnation of such falsehoods, but accept them as perfectly natural. Only in that way can the full truth be discovered. And it is vitally important that as much of the truth about every case should be obtained and studied. It is true that the venereal diseases are physical afflictions, and once they have been identified treatment can be prescribed without reference to other factors. Yet the background provides essential data for getting to know how these diseases are spread; and the more we know about that, the more surely we can make our plans for controlling their dissemination.

'I know I've been a ruddy fool,' he said shamefacedly, 'and I hope I'm not making things worse by wasting your time.'

'The only thing that interests me,' I replied, 'is that you have exposed yourself to a serious risk of infection, and so far from being a "ruddy fool" as you put it, you are in fact an extremely wise young man to come and see me. If, as you say, there are no signs, that makes you all the wiser, for few would trouble to come in those circumstances. I wish everyone showed as much commonsense.'

'Well, you see,' he said looking very relieved at my attitude, 'I don't suppose I'd be in such a flap if it wasn't for Diana and the baby. There – there's no risk she's been infected, is there, as I've no chancre or anything?'

'I wish I could say "no",' I answered. 'We can't answer that question till we've found out whether you're infected or not. You say all this happened about three to four weeks ago?'

'Yes,' he nodded.

'Then the absence of any external sign isn't at all abnormal assuming you've been infected. The usual period is between ten and twenty-one days, but it's been known to appear in nine days and sometimes there's no chancre till three months have elapsed. But we'll have to have you tested.'

'Very well, doctor,' he said. 'And Diana? Will she have to be tested too?'

This is one of the taut moments in these interviews – when the husband has to be made to realize that he must not leave his wife in ignorance any longer.

'At the moment,' I said, 'the principal thing is to find out what state you're in. If there's infection, then, of course, your wife will have to know and will have to be examined.'

'Let's hope she hadn't got it,' he exclaimed fervently.

'I'm afraid I shall have to speak very seriously about that,' I said, knowing that it is better to bring patients face to face with the truth as soon as possible so as to give them no chance of harbouring illusory hopes. 'In your case, I shall recommend that, whatever the results of these first tests, your wife shall come to me.'

He opened his eyes in surprise. 'But doctor ...' he began.

'It's the only course,' I insisted. 'It is quite possible that these first tests on you may be negative. That doesn't mean that I can say you're not infected. In some cases tests may be carried out over months before we discover the infection beyond doubt – though that's comparatively rare. But against that must be set the fact that in this primary stage, the infectivity, as we say, that is, the power of transmitting disease to others – is extremely high; in your case that means that the danger to your wife is very high.'

'I see,' he said slowly. The look of dull anxiety in his eyes is one with which I have grown only too familiar.

'And your wife is pregnant. That is the overriding reason. Even if we were to get negative results on tests on your wife, I should still insist on her undergoing treatment to protect the unborn child. The horrors of congenital syphilis or even gonorrhoea are so terrible that no precaution is too great.'

To this he returned no answer. He stared broodingly at the floor. I agreed with his probable thoughts; that this was surely too heavy a price to pay for a single night's folly. But I did not expect him to protest or try to evade the issue. He had shown so much wisdom so far that he would not retreat at the last step. Nor was I mistaken.

'Yes, I shall have to tell her,' he said slowly but decisively. 'I think I shall feel better in any case getting on the level with Diana.'

'That's a very sensible attitude,' I remarked. 'It's the only possible one. I'm sure you wouldn't want to buy a little peace now at the cost of being responsible for bringing an infected child into the world, and I'm also sure that there's nothing you wouldn't do to prevent that.'

'Nothing,' he said with a sigh.

I took a blood sample. It was all I could do, since there was no lesion from which to extract serum for examination. This meant that, in all probability, some little time must elapse before I could give this worried young patient a definite ruling. The Wassermann test of the blood very often remains negative for as long as eight weeks after infection, and the first diagnosis is, as a rule, made by the identification of the spirochaete in the fluid drawn from the initial chancre. This is done by means of the dark-ground microscope, an adaptation of the normal instrument which shows the organism against a black background instead of a bright one.

There would be a further delaying factor if no overt clinical evidence appeared in the form of a chancre or other sign. It is usual in such cases to postpone treatment until the Wassermann reaction has remained consistently positive for about three months. But in this case, I certainly would not do so. If there were the slightest suspicion I should advise immediate treatment for himself and his wife; the child was too valuable to run risks even of the remotest sort. I sent him away with instructions to return the next day.

'Shall I bring Diana?' he asked anxiously.

In view of the circumstances, I very nearly said 'yes'; but I decided to let him have time to get over what I was sure was going to be a very difficult ordeal for him. 'No,' I said. 'Not this time. We won't run ahead too fast.'

He shot me a grateful glance and departed.

As I rather expected, the test was negative. His case was urgent – not for himself but because of the possible effects on his wife and her unborn child, and I seriously considered administering the 'provocative' injection of neoarsphenamine. When the Wassermann test is negative, an injection of this drug which is, of course, used in the treatment of syphilis, will often promote or 'provoke' a positive reaction. It is, however, not usual to resort to this measure until sufficient time has elapsed for the Wassermann test to give an informative reaction, and, in Christopher's case, this period was barely past. Moreover, there was still a chance that a chancre might develop, in which event we would be on surer ground, but the injection of neoarsphenamine might retard or even inhibit its development. I decided to wait a little while longer, and in the meantime carry out routine-newer and more sensitive tests. Perhaps Christopher was not infected at all! Even a pessimistic doctor is allowed to hope for the better.

There was one point here that had, perhaps, better be explained. It might seem strange to treat this case as one of suspected syphilis in the complete absence of any direct evidence – and also to rule out the possibility that if an infection was present it might be the other chief venereal disease – gonorrhoea. But this is the course the doctor must always adopt. In VD treatment it is the absolute rule that the suspect must be regarded as guilty till he is proved innocent. As to gonorrhoea as a possibility, it could be dismissed for all practical purposes, in Christopher's case, for by this time there would have been abundant signs of its presence.

Two days after I had made the third routine examination – this time with more sensitive tests – Christopher returned to me in great alarm. He had observed a small 'spot', as he termed it, on his genital organs. In the normal course of events, he would probably not have noticed it so soon, but under my instructions, he was examining himself closely and continually. I think its appearance had shattered the hopes which, in spite of all my warnings, he had allowed himself to build up on the repeated negative reactions of the tests. It is such quite understandable hopes that lead a large number of patients to discontinue their periodical tests; they feel that the doctor is being over-cautious, whereas, as a matter of fact, it is impossible to exercise too much caution in these cases. Perhaps in no type of treatment (except again in psychiatry) is so much co-operation demanded of the patient as in these stages of suspended judgement of venereal disease.

I took a careful look at the 'spot'. To the experienced eye, a syphilitic chancre, even when it has just erupted, is almost unmistakable. Almost at sight, I felt that here was the definite confirmation that it is always distressing to see. Distressing – yes, in the sense that it is always tragic to have to advise a patient that he has contracted infection and must submit to treatment; and yet in many ways it is a relief. One knows where one stands and the anxious period of uncertainty is over.

Christopher, I knew, shared that view to some extent; he was anxious to know one way or the other, and the continued strain of waiting was having a bad effect on him psychologically. I determined, therefore, to make an immediate Darkfield examination of the pus from the lesion. This is a fairly rapid procedure when one has had some experience of it. It was not long, therefore, before I knew definitely.

'I'm afraid,' I said gravely, "that the worst has been confirmed. Of course, even the presence of the spirochaetes in the fluid is not, by itself, proof positive, but I think it is sufficient for action. You agree we can't take the slightest risk. Certainly, I shall have to see your wife now.'

He nodded slowly as though in confirmation of his own thoughts. It was the first time I had referred to that aspect of the case directly since our initial conversation. Until I had something definite to go upon I could not take a strong line. As to whether he thought it advisable to discuss the matter with his wife, and so prepare her for what might have to be, that rested on him alone meanwhile. I hoped he had.

'That's a blow,' he remarked dejectedly. 'I'd begun to allow myself a little hope. But she knows. She took it marvellously, and she's quite ready. No one could have backed me up better.' He paused for a moment. 'It was a horrible job, but it did relieve me a lot to talk to her. All right, I'll bring her along.'

I found Diana a charming, co-operative, and realistic patient. But she had had some hospital experience as a nurse and had none of that ingrained objection to medical treatment of any kind which some women seem to possess. She did not say very much, but it was easy to see that the whole affair had come as a terrible shock to her – as well it might.

Practically the only certainty about syphilis is its uncertainty. One very, very rarely – I had almost said never – meets, even in a wide experience, two cases that are exactly alike. And these two cases, though both presumably infected by spirochaetes of exactly the same strain showed marked differences. As a general rule, the effect of the venereal diseases in general, and markedly so in syphilis, are less severe in the female patient than in the male, though in both the final upshot of untreated disease is equally tragic. Yet here we had Christopher presenting difficulties in diagnosis while his wife, Diana, was a practically obvious case from the moment of first examination. The chancre was well developed, and the Darkfield test gave an immediate positive finding, as did the Wassermann test. Christopher did not react positively to the latter till his next examination.

Again, as I wanted to be as certain as I could, I used the combined penicillin and neoarsphenamine treatment, although slightly outmoded and by some doctors discarded at the present time. Both responded well, and the secondary stage was not marked in either – though curiously, it was again Diana who had the more severe symptoms.

They came together for the tests after the course of treatment was over, and on one occasion they obviously had something to say to me.

'Tell me, doctor,' said Diana, 'I know you can't say definitely yet that either of us is cured, but I suppose by taking it in time like this the baby will be quite safe now?'

She looked at me anxiously. I wished I could have replied with an unambiguous affirmative.

'That is more than I or anyone can say,' I replied. 'This is something I've been meaning to tell you for some time. You have done all you can and I would go so far as to say that the probabilities are that your child will be absolutely free from infection and without any external signs – stigmata as we call them – of congenital disease. But there are certain things that are absolutely essential. You must bring the baby to me soon after it is born, so that I can examine it thoroughly – and again after about a year, say. That is a vital precaution. And more than that you must not fail to consult me or any other clinic wherever you may be, if there is the slightest suspicion of anything wrong in later years. I am giving you the blackest side of the picture but I think you will agree that it is better for me to do so.'

'Yes, doctor,' she said in a low strained voice. 'But what does that mean? Can't you say definitely whether baby will be free or not?'

I shook my head. 'No', I replied. 'That is the tragedy of it. The tests may be negative and continue negative, and then, when the child is growing up and you've almost forgotten all about it, it suddenly develops some of the signs of late syphilis. The disease is known as latent congenital syphilis.'

'All the same,' I went on, 'there's not the slightest need to dwell on that aspect of the case. I'm only telling you what *might* happen as a remote contingency. My opinion is that the chances of anything of the sort happening are so slight that you need not worry beyond keeping the possibility at the back of your minds. I believe that penicillin clears everything up completely, and the only reason I can't say so definitely is because we have no records yet of penicillin-treated cases after the lapse of several years. In time, we shall, and then it won't in my view be necessary for doctors to say things I've just been forced to say.'

'Thank you, doctor,' she said. 'You've been wonderful to us both all along. I don't know how we can ever thank you enough. If ... if' – she hesitated as though the words were difficult to say – my baby should show any signs, I'm absolutely certain that it won't be through any fault of yours, but only because luck is dead against us both.'

'That's very nice of you,' I replied. 'But don't thank me. If you wish to thank anyone, thank your husband. If it hadn't been for his consideration of and love for you and his quite uncommon sense in coming to me on no more than a slight suspicion, the case might have been different.'

She smiled at me, and the smile overflowed to Christopher, who looked a little confused.

In due course the baby was born – as healthy and vigorous a boy as any parents could desire. My examinations have revealed nothing that could give rise to the slightest suspicions of congenital syphilis, and with the mounting experience of penicillin and with other antibiotics treatment, I do not think he ever will reveal any. Miracle of miracles, Christopher and Diana have adopted me as a personal friend and appointed me an honorary and brevet Uncle to young Norman. There are very few people who care to claim the acquaintance of a venereal-disease specialist for fear of unworthy suspicions, such is the state of the public mind!

These two people are happy. Yet how different it might all have turned out!

How easy it would have been for Christopher to persuade himself that he had run no risk at all – and easier still to postpone treatment till the worst had happened. For little Norman was never infected at all, thanks to treatment in time. A little later, and the damage might have been done. True, we could have cured the baby, as we can most cases today, except for a few that have remained untreated for many years, but it is better never to have been infected at all.

I may possibly see Diana again – as a patient. That does not sound any sort of compliment to my treatment or faith in myself or my drugs. If she comes, it will be because she is a wise woman who abhors exposing the innocent to risks and suffering. She will come if she is going to have another baby, as she hopes one day to do. Then I shall give her another course of treatment to guard against any infection that may still, as the remotest of chances, be lurking in her system. Once again, I believe that when we know more about penicillin and the other wonderful antibiotic drugs, we shall no longer need to give this advice. But until we do, it is a precaution that every pregnant woman who has once been treated for venereal disease of any kind should take. To make assurance doubly sure, to eliminate the merest hint of risk, is the least one can do for a life as yet unborn.

Case 6

BETTY

Behind almost every case of venereal disease lies a tragedy – or the materials for a tragedy. I am not now thinking of the immediate physical effects; what I have in mind are the tragedies of ignorance, superstition, weakness, and crass folly, that go to the making of these cases. In a sense, I suppose, that is true of a great deal of human suffering, much of which could be avoided if the devils of ignorance and superstition and weakness and folly did not have, as it seems, a permanent home in the human personality. But in the VD Clinic one becomes acutely aware of the monsters, for it is part of the physician's duty to discover all he can of the history of each case, to trace back to its origins the cause of the disease. This is something that never, for me at least, loses its poignancy. It is not so much that each case is different; it is rather the similarities underlying the superficial differences that make one sad – at times despondent; for it is precisely this which indicates how human beings, for seemingly good reasons, for obviously bad reasons, and often for no reason at all, will go on repeating the same pattern of error.

There was Betty's case, for example – though, strictly speaking it was Pearl's case first of all. Betty's history is, in its general outlines, very much too familiar, and it raises deep and perplexing problems that lie at the roots of modern civilization and are of wider significance even than the prevention of venereal disease and the arrest of its dissemination.

As I have said, it was Pearl's case first of all – though I doubt very much whether my patient had officially had that name conferred on her when she was brought to me. For Pearl was then three days old. She was the daughter of a woman who had been admitted to the Maternity Department to have her child – that was all I was at the time – and when the baby was three days old it showed marked signs of inflammation round the eyes and eyelids. It was sent to me for examination.

There is a condition known as 'ophthalmia neonatorum' – ophthalmia or eye affliction of the newborn – which is regarded very seriously in every civilised country, and if its signs and symptoms, which include inflammation of the eyes and a purulent discharge, make their appearance within twenty-one days of birth, the condition must be notified at once to the district Medical Officer of Health.

Strictly speaking, ophthalmia neonatorum is not a single disease or condition; several states answer to the definition which is, really, nothing more than a convenient portmanteau expression. But it is right that this strict precaution, failure to obey which may involve heavy penalties and fines for continued failure to report, should be observed, for one of the most common causes of the condition is the gonococcus – the germ which causes the other important venereal disease – gonorrhoea. If this type of infection is demonstrated in the child suffering from ophthalmia neonatorum, it establishes beyond all doubt that the mother is a victim of gonorrhoea, and that the child has been infected at the time of delivery. That is why in the eyes of every newborn baby drops of antiseptics – in recent years drops of antibiotic solutions – are put so that the danger of infection is minimised as much as possible.

This is one striking difference between syphilis and gonorrhoea, so far as the diseases are transmittable from mother to her children. In syphilis the spirochaete invades the unborn child from the mother's blood stream; the child may thus become syphilitic while it is still in its mother's womb. But in gonorrhoea, should the mother become pregnant, no such invasion occurs. The gonococcus reaches the child during the actual process of birth by coming into contact with the infected part of the mother's body. It is an important difference in many ways, but one of the most practical points is that if a gonorrhoeal mother takes treatment during pregnancy and is cured, there is no risk of infecting the child when it is born, while on the other hand, the offspring of a syphilitic mother is likely to be infected at birth despite the mother having taken treatment successfully, and it must, therefore, undergo curative measures itself.

Pearl, then, was brought to my department when she was three days old and we had no difficulties in establishing the existence of the gonococcus in the discharge from the inflamed eyes. The child's eyelids were red and swollen and had already developed a slightly glazed appearance, while being hot to the touch. Luckily we were able to place her under penicillin treatment, both locally and by injections, the effect of which is almost dramatic in this type of case, at the outset, for if allowed to go untreated ophthalmia neonatorum can lead to dire results on the cornea of the eyes and complete loss of sight. Treatment cannot be given too soon. In bad cases of heavy infection – mercifully very rare these days – the cornea – the transparent sheath of the eye – may be perforated within twenty-four to thirty-six hours, with the high probability of complete blindness and the practical certainty of impaired vision throughout life if the great evil is averted. So it is obvious that action must be prompt and effective. As to the first, the law tries to enforce it by its insistence, under heavy penalty, of instant notification; as to the latter, modern methods of treatment, notably penicillin and other more recent antibiotics, are completely successful.

The baby's case, then, was completely simple in the medical sense, and it presented no difficulties in the event. Since the case was being handled in the Clinic, we were able to arrange for the baby to be separated from its mother, for though reinfection was unlikely to cause a recurrence of the eye trouble, there is another condition, known as vulvo-vaginitis which may affect children who make contact with the gonococcus. There remained the mother. She must obviously be infected with gonorrhoea, and I speculated on what sort of woman she be who allowed herself to remain untreated for gonorrhoea throughout her pregnancy.

I soon found out; and the story, by no means as unusual as might be thought, forms a somewhat sordid sidelight on our social conditions. The first thing that struck me was that Betty the mother, did not seem unduly distressed about the narrowly averted disaster to her child; the second one was that she seemed sullen and puzzled about it. Indeed her manner was almost resentful, as though she considered she was being submitted to a degradation for no reason whatsoever. And that attitude made it very difficult to obtain from her a reliable story of the background to the case. There was no doubt that she was suffering from gonorrhoea. More than that, it had remained untreated for a long time.

Once again, penicillin, the miracle-worker, was called into action. She was kept in hospital for forty-eight hours and given the maximum dosage. As a rule, hospitalization for forty-four hours is sufficient for the treatment of gonorrhoea by penicillin, but as in this case the welfare of the child was at stake, I decided that it was better to leave nothing to chance. After that, of course, the regular routine examinations and tests came to make sure that the cure was complete – first, at weekly intervals, then at monthly ones, and finally at three months' periods, the whole covering one year.

In view of her resentment and moroseness over the whole affair, I was quite expecting to find that she would soon give up coming to the Clinic for examination, but in this I was mistaken. She paid her visits with unfailing regularity, and it was during the progress of these that I managed to piece together the sequence of events that had led up to her infection.

It was a melancholy enough tale. Betty's mother had died while she was still very young, and she had been brought up by a father who had little interest in her and took his parental responsibilities with far less seriousness than his loyalty to the local publican. Perhaps to rid himself of what duties still obtruded themselves on him, though he enlisted in the Army, and was sent to a depot in Scotland. At the immature age of fifteen, Betty was left to fend for herself.

The prospect did not alarm her; she was used to being her own mistress. In fact, she said, it was a relief, for now she had only herself to look after and her wages were her own. Since she had left school and become a wage-earner in a factory, her father had come to look on her pay if not as a prop of the home, at any rate as a useful additional source of drinking money. He had not scrupled to demand practically everything, even resorting to threats and actual violence if he considered them the only way of getting what he wanted. As might have been expected, Betty had a shrewd head. She sold up the remains of the family home in the small provincial town where she had spent the whole of her short and not very pleasant life, came to London, and secured a job at a good wage in a factory.

The sequel was commonplace enough – though it is not a very reassuring commentary on our attitude nowadays that we are prepared to accept it as commonplace. With her lack of normal upbringing and her preoccupation with self-interest, she became an easy victim of laxity of the post-war years. It was all too easy for a girl with no particular standards of self-discipline to have a 'good time', and Betty who, till then, had known practically nothing of good times of any kind grasped the opportunity with both hands.

Of course, the inevitable happened; she soon found that she was going to have a baby; and it was impossible for her to say who the father might have been. By that time she had progressed far in what is sometimes called worldly wisdom. She did not want to be embarrassed by a baby especially as she was only nineteen and the opportunities for good times seemed to be increasing rather than decreasing. It was not a difficult matter to arrange for the child – a boy – to be taken care of and later someone might care to adopt him. But even in his absence, the baby still proved a burden. His board and so on had to be paid for; and Betty was growing reluctant to work. The whole business, in her eyes, was deplorable. Still, wages were good, and the favours she granted so easily were not without their money value – though she would have resented hotly any suggestion that she was a professional.

Gradually matters began to grow really difficult. She had not heard at all from her father, and she did not care if she never had news of him again. She did not want his help anyway. But it was not easy to earn money, and certainly the plethora of good times was passing. The factory at which she worked closed; the idea of looking for a new job repelled her. There was still the child to keep; and so, like so many others, she dropped her amateur status and took to the streets professionally.

Realization that she was going to have a second child came as a severe shock to her; she regarded it as the work of a particularly malign fate.

'I never thought I'd get caught a second time,' she said bitterly, 'and I don't know how I slipped up. After all, I was only a kid the first time. Of course, I tried all the usual things to get rid of it.'

I smiled very grimly. 'Of course,' she had said, as though all these quack remedies and traditional herbs were still worth trying to put an end to an unwanted pregnancy. It is amazing – and appalling – how strongly superstition will hold even in the face of failure after failure. And that was how she came originally to the Clinic.

In the end, she had gone to try her luck with an abortionist. My gorge rises when I think of these men and women who attempt to terminate pregnancies under conditions that would make even a hygiene worker, let alone a surgeon, shudder, and whose qualifications are nothing more than an ability to inspire credulous and often desperate women with an illusory confidence. To make it worse, Betty's was almost a full term pregnancy – Pearl was an eight-month baby when she was born. No wonder that most of the doctors today, and a great majority of our citizen welcome with open hearts the new law that allows abortions to be performed by qualified and well trained medical men in properly equipped clinics. We, doctors, know how much unhappiness and misery has been spared these unfortunate women, not to speak of how many lives have been saved in the process, by this enlightened and humane law.

In Betty's case, the criminal's activities seem to have been more than usually disastrous, though she was careful never to divulge the smallest detail about the person's sex or address. She was rushed to the Clinic as an emergency case. So, from a background of squalor, little Pearl came into the world with the seeds of tragedy in her own innocent body.

'But surely you must have known you were infected?' I asked her.

She shook her head. 'Why should I?' she demanded.

'Well, you've been running risks for a long time,' I pointed out. 'Didn't you ever suspect it?'

She shrugged. 'Maybe once or twice,' she answered, as though it was of only passing consequence. 'But why should I worry? It didn't interfere with me much anyway, and in any event it was only clap.'

'Why didn't you go to a clinic and make sure?' I asked. 'Apart from yourself, didn't you mind possibly infecting other people?'

Her eyes brightened and she curled her lips. 'Go to one of those places and get a pi-jaw on the evil of my life? Not me! And why should I care about giving it to someone else? If men go with me, they do it with their eyes open, and they've only themselves to blame if they get a dose. They're usually too tight to worry anyhow. And, as we are on the subject, what about the man who gave the disease to me? Was he worried also?'

I sighed softly. 'And even when you knew you were going to have a baby and that all these efforts you were making to get rid of it would probably be unsuccessful, you still didn't think it worth while to have an examination for the child's sake?'

She looked at me as though I made a completely astonishing statement.

'How the hell was I to know it'd affect the kid?' she demanded quite offended. 'I knew pox did, but not this.'

'Well,' I said, 'you know now. And you also know that you've probably infected quite a few men, who've gone back to their wives and infected them and quite possibly some of their babies.'

Again she shrugged as if it was no concern of hers.

It is not a part of my duty or my purpose to express any sort of judgement on her. Even if it were, could I or anyone condemn her as wholly bad? If we condemn her, do we not also and more strongly condemn ourselves as the members of a society that makes it so easy for girls to tread the path she trod? What is more important to me is the ignorance she revealed and the mass of misconception to which she subscribed.

There is some justification for her when she said she did not know she had gonorrhoea, for in a woman it is often difficult to detect, and the overt symptoms are slight and easily confused with manifestations of other kinds. So far we can go with her, though no further. Take her points one by one. 'It was only clap,' she said, dismissing, by its vulgar name, gonorrhoea as a minor disease of no particular importance. That is a very wide-spread belief, yet how wrong it is! True, its results are not so spectacular as those of syphilis can be, Nevertheless, if untreated, gonorrhoea can have far-reaching and almost crippling effects on the human body, notably in widespread 'rheumatic' pains and more terrible, in deterioration and sometimes loss of sight.

She would not go to a clinic because she did not want to have a 'pi-jaw on the evil of my young life.' It took me a long time, in those interviews, to gain her confidence and make her believe I was not going to sit in judgement on her. Yet the attitude is a reflection of still too prevalent belief that venereal diseases are mixed up everywhere with morals and cannot be regarded solely as a medical problem. If that young woman had had – shall we say – acne or diphtheria or even a chronic catarrh, she would almost certainly have gone to the doctor. But because she faintly suspected gonorrhoea, she held back, fearing the disease less than the moral obloquy she expected.

Her indifference to the fate of the men who were her clients is partly personal idiosyncrasy, for which, going outside my own sphere, I think there is a psychological explanation though I will not pursue that here. But also – and this is important – it is a condemnation of a system that breeds young people with no sense of responsibility to their fellows and fails to tell them the plain, unvarnished truth about the venereal diseases.

So, too with her continued indifference when she knew she was to have a baby. Here again it is ignorance and misinformation that led her to think that only syphilis could infect a child – a belief that far, far too many people hold. Note also the indifference in her attitude towards the quacks and abortionists to whom she resorted, on the one hand, and towards VD clinics and doctors on the other. The former, for all their dangers, offered possible help without questions asked; the latter might help – but only at the expense of condemnation. VD clinics it would seem, were not so much medical institutions as part and parcel of the system of organized conventional morals, from which she was an outcast and for which they would seek to reclaim her. It is that dangerous, disastrous confusion which is so hard to kill. The difference of attitude is none the less significant because it is implied in her statements and not openly expressed. Again we can be grateful that these attitudes are slowly but surely changing for the better.

I pressed Betty hard in an attempt to discover how long she had had the disease. Obviously, it was of some fair standing. Leading questions had to be put to her for the very adequate reasons that she was ignorant of all except the grossest signs of gonorrhoea.

At last I managed to fix the date at which she had first noticed a slight discharge – usually the most significant and suspicious indication – at about two to two-and-a-half years earlier. But it had been accompanied by none of the other signs, so far as she could remember at that length of time. Obviously, if they had been there, they must have been slight. Yet this is not so very uncommon in women, for gonorrhoea and syphilis alike tend to be less acute in the female than in the male, and so far as actual inflammations or lesions in the genital organs are concerned, they are very much less likely to be noticed in the woman than in the man. She confessed to having had 'some sort of rheumatism' for a year or perhaps more. It was not associated with any particular region but the pain had seemed to shift from joint to joint. In her examination I had established the fact of diffuse arthralgia due to infection by the gonococcus. This is a fairly frequent result of long-standing gonorrhoea, though similar states that imitate the various kinds of what is popularly called rheumatism and neuritis often occur.

There could be no thought, in Betty's case, of trying to trace down the source of infection with a view of trying to eliminate it. The facts were rather that she herself had been the active source of infection of probably a good many male cases. And even if she had gone to a clinic at the first faint suspicions, it would no doubt have been difficult to single out any one particular man as the originator of her disease, in view of the life she had led.

My task was ended when I was able to tell her that her examinations now showed that there were no gonococci present in her. That is the farthest one can go; the bacteriologist will never say more than that he can find no evidence of the gonococcus. I warned her, too, that if ever she became pregnant again, she must go at once to a clinic for examination and possible treatment in the interest of her child.

'I'll watch it,' she said sullenly. 'I'm not getting caught again. After this packet I'd rather chuck myself into the Thames. All the same, if it should happen, I'll come to you.'

'The nearest clinic will give you attention quite as good,' I said, not wishing to give her any excuse.

'No,' she insisted, shaking her head firmly, 'you or no one.'

I knew what she meant. Personally, I proved to her that she would get no lectures or sermons; I had won her confidence by the clear absence, on my part, of any desire to pluck a brand from the burning. Yet I had not succeeded in completely dispelling from her mind that most people, including doctors in VD clinics in general, associate venereal diseases with morals and look on sufferers as outcasts. Well, she is unfortunately right as regards some members of the public, including not a few who ought to know better. But she is wrong about doctors at large and VD doctors in particular – and that is something which cannot be too widely known.

But something at least has been gained. She is cured herself. Her baby is safe ... And a potential source of infection has, for the time being at least (on a pessimistic view), been cleared up. She has, too, received quite a lot of enlightenment which may save her more mistakes, not least in that she is now thoroughly scared of the dangers of gonorrhoea no less than of syphilis. She told me nothing of her plans, for she is of habit, a secretive woman who resents intrusion into her affairs. None the less she informed the Almoner that she did not wish to take steps to have the baby adopted. Perhaps Betty has learnt her lesson. Let us hope she has.

But if she has, ought she and her baby to have paid the whole of the price? Is it right that you and I and the fifty-odd-million other inhabitants of Great Britain should pass by on the other side?

Case 7

SON AND FATHER

One of the most encouraging signs of the times to a venereal diseases specialist is the decline of cases of congenital syphilis during recent years. To many who have been shocked by widespread talk of an increase in venereal disease due to so-called 'general moral laxity' – an increase which official statistics seem to support – this decrease in congenital syphilis may seem surprising and paradoxical. That it is real cannot be doubted.

Many cases have contributed to it and continue to do so. There is, for example, the wonderful improvement in the prenatal maternity services which has been effected in the past decade or so. Infected mothers who might otherwise have done nothing about their condition have been passed to the VD clinics for treatment during pregnancy, and thus the chance of their having perfectly healthy offspring has been very considerably increased. Wider knowledge of the facts of venereal disease is, too, inducing more and more victims to make use voluntarily of the free and highly efficient services of the public clinics.

As to the apparent contradiction between the general statistics for venereal diseases and the decline in the incidence of congenital syphilis, it must never be forgotten that statistics by themselves give little useful information. They can, in fact, be positively misleading. It is true that the members of those attending for the first time at VD clinics and found to be infected has shown a rise, but this does not, of course, indicate that the rate of incidence of new disease is rising. On the contrary, one undoubted reason for the rise in the number of cases is the slowly improving awareness of the public to the dangers of venereal disease; a higher proportion of cases come to the clinics. There is no means of ascertaining with certainty the extent of venereal disease among the population as a whole, but there is ample evidence to show that the willingness to have treatment is far greater today than ever before – though still not so high as it should and must be made. Thus it is even possible – though not perhaps probable – that over the population as a whole, venereal disease is less rife today than at any previous time, the much higher proportion of sufferers coming to the clinics giving the impression that the overall incidence is rising. These are crucial facts that must never be forgotten – especially by those who seek to draw moral inferences and teach moral lessons on the basis of unqualified, crude medical statistics.

But if there is this improvement, it does not mean that the curse of congenital syphilis is anything like being on the point of extermination. There are still too many people who are prepared to remain untreated and whose carelessness and ignorance are a higher danger to the health of the community as a whole. If only their own welfare was concerned, one might be justified in shrugging one's shoulders, and saying that, if they prefer ill-health and often actual suffering with probably worse to come, then they are entitled to the life of their choice. But it is not so. Every untreated syphilitic is a social menace, either active or retrospective and, as such, cannot be taken lightly or permitted to indulge his own anti-social proclivities.

Today then, the field of congenital syphilis is one that, to me at least, gives the most cause for restrained hope. If syphilis is itself increasing (and again I stress that it is impossible to say one way or the other) then I believe that it is more than offset by the high efficaciousness of contemporary therapy. Thus, the chances of a child being born syphilitic steadily decrease. I do not think that this is an exaggerated picture, for I am not at all inclined to minimize the generally unsatisfactory position in the fight against the venereal diseases. It is, however, only right to point out a lightening of the sky where it can be discerned.

None the less many cases of congenital syphilis do occur. Some of the most remarkable are those of late, or delayed, disease in which the victim appears suddenly to develop the signs and symptoms of the tertiary stage. Congenital syphilis is termed 'late' when it shows itself at any age after two years. When it delays its appearance till after the twentieth year, which although uncommon, is not by any means a striking rarity, it has a special name, Lues tarda.

The case of Harold was a most interesting one of congenital syphilis, not merely in itself but also for the circumstances surrounding it. Apart from all else, it does show that, even today, it is possible for congenital syphilis to be overlooked and the small signs ignored in the slow, almost imperceptible, progress of the affliction.

Harold was sent to me with a note from the Army medical authorities. He was eighteen, had enlisted and had presented himself for the medical examination. The examining doctor had taken one look at him and made up his mind, as he had every justification in doing, for Harold was an almost perfect picture of late congenital syphilis, showing many of the classical stigmata, and subsequent Wassemann tests gave the expected confirmation of the clinical diagnosis.

Before going on to deal with the features of Harold's individual case, let us try to get a few things clear about congenital syphilis – about which, as about all the venereal diseases, so many misconceptions and even superstitions exist.

First of all, then, it is congenital and not hereditary – that is to say it is not transmitted from the father or mother by way of the germ plasm of the sex cells, as true hereditary characters are, like eye colour, for example. A syphilitic father cannot have a syphilitic child without first infecting the mother, from whose infected blood the embryo acquires the disease. In the early days of syphilitic treatment, failure to recognize this fact led to a great deal of confusion and worse.

Secondly, when syphilis does not reveal itself early – that is, before the age of two years – it often has no obvious effect on the development of the child. It is true that it can have the most terrible results on a young child, sometimes producing babies that look like wizened old men and women. But in the majority of cases of congenital syphilis these gross deformities are not present. The child grows up naturally, seemingly perfectly healthy and in no way different from its fellows. In congenital syphilis, too, the primary stage of chancre is absent; early cases are typical of the secondary stage, sometimes so slight that they pass unnoticed. It will be recalled that the secondary stage in acquired syphilis is often almost signless and symptomless, and this asymptomatic condition, as it is called, is particularly prevalent when the disease is congenital.

Late congenital syphilis, which may occur at any age, though most often before the twentieth year, reveals itself by the sudden development of symptoms of the tertiary stage. In certain cases it might, indeed, be confused with the tertiary stage of acquired syphilis, but for some very remarkable phenomena which are peculiar to the congenital variety.

Simply put, the sequence of events has been this. While the disease has been without symptoms (asymptomatic) the spirochaetes have been doing their evil work in secret within the body. Certain structures fail to develop normally – among them the teeth – while others, having grown more or less as in the healthy ·child, become infected or deformed. As to the latter, the results of spirochaete infection are often only detectable by X-ray photographs. When the evidence of disease finally come out into the open, it is as though a long-smouldering fire has suddenly burst into flame.

A congenital syphilitic with all the stigmata of his condition presents an absolutely unmistakable picture – the one case of venereal disease that can be diagnosed with practical certainty almost at a glance. The face is particularly noticeable, for it tends to become dish-shaped, while the nose is bridgeless resulting in the often depicted 'saddle nose'. Beetling brows are another feature, but this is due less to actual deformity of structure than to the fact that the sufferer has eye trouble and thus contracts a habit of pulling the brows down to reduce the painful effect of light.

The Army medical officer examining Harold, as I have said, recognized his condition at once, but I should not describe the boy as a really gross example of congenital syphilis. There was enough about him to make the diagnosis obvious, but none of the stigmata had been carried to extremes. All the same, for anyone wishing to see what effect congenital syphilis can have on a growing human being, his case is well worth a little description.

His face was noticeably flat or dish-shaped (it is difficult to describe this appearance in words, but it is instantly recognizable) though the expression was distinctly what is known so vividly in modern slang as 'dumb'. The bridge of the nose was markedly underdeveloped, but not to the point of making a saddle nose; rather was it slightly concave. The eyebrows were pulled down a little and the lids tended to droop so that he gave the appearance of looking at one through half-closed eyes.

Diagnosis of all kinds is a cumulative process. One sign or symptom by itself may indicate a dozen possible states, but taken in conjunction with others, its particular meaning in each case becomes clear. The combination of signs and symptoms gives what is known as the clinical picture of the condition. So it was with Harold. Each one of the signs I have mentioned might be due to other states than congenital syphilis, yet taken together they raised a very strong suspicion indeed.

This suspicion was confirmed the further one looked for the tell-tale stigmata. First of all, having taken a general look at him, I examined his teeth, paying particular attention to the incisors – the front cutting teeth – and to the first molars – the 'double teeth'. Here again the stigmata were developed, not, it is true, to a very marked extent but sufficiently to leave no doubt to the experienced eye. Congenital syphilis produces what are known as Hutchinson's incisors; the teeth tend to become shaped like a barrel or a tapering wedge, with the narrowest part at the cutting edge which itself is notched. This is one of the most important stigmata, and so far as Harold was concerned, there could be no doubt whatever. The molars had the appearance of small domes. What happens is that the normal cusps of the grinding teeth are underdeveloped and disappear rapidly from the combined effects of decay and wear, leaving, in place of the normally shaped tooth, a simple dome, often with a surface that looks, on close examination, rather like a honeycomb. These are called 'Moon's molars'.

Harold's mouth had been disgracefully neglected. Apart from the stigmata of syphilis, there was widespread decay, and I could not help wondering how any person could have gone about with his teeth in such condition. There, incidentally, lies another reason why, today, congenital syphilis is sooner recognized and dealt with. Any competent dentist would have seen what was the matter with Harold and suggested the need for proper attention. The wider care today for teeth is responsible for many boons beside the obvious one of a sound mouth.

The examination of a case of congenital syphilis has to be even more searching than of one of acquired disease, for there is scarcely a structure or organ of the body that may not be affected in some way. The bones and joints, the eyes, and the ears, are perhaps the parts most commonly involved, but in the later stages neuro-syphilis may develop – the condition that leads in the end to what is popularly known as general paralysis of the insane or GPI, though the term more usually used today by doctors is general paresis. The heart, arteries, veins, intestines and other organs may also become infected. All of these states may, of course, arise also in acquired syphilis, but there is a higher probability of their appearing in the congenital variety for the simple reason that the sufferer more often than not does not suspect his condition.

Harold, then, had some of the most typical stigmata of congenital syphilis as regards the teeth, and others were also present, as I quickly discovered. There was slight deafness, due to the infection of the nerves of the inner ear. His eyes looked dull and slightly opaque, rather like an opal without the fiery iridescence of the gem-eyes that fully answered Shakespeare's adjective of 'lack-lustre'. His sight was a good way beneath normal vision and he also exhibited some degree of photophobia – a tendency to avoid light, because its incidence on the eye causes discomfort or even pain.

Not unexpectedly he complained of having experienced, from time to time, shifting pain in the joints. He had, however, only one of the typical stigmata in this connection – a slight development of what are known as Clutton's joints. There are swellings at the knee joints that sometimes become so enlarged as to make walking difficult. X-ray photographs show no abnormalities in the bone structure itself, the condition being due to a form of syphilitic tumour – a gumma – in the joint. Harold's knees had not enlarged to the point of interference with his gait, apart from a slight tendency to walk straddle-legged, and there was no pain; there never is any attached to this affliction.

Routine Wassermann and other serological tests gave the confirmation of what was already certain. Harold's state was due to congenital syphilis. He was put under treatment, and after combined penicillin and arsenotherapy he showed marked improvement. Treatment of congenital syphilis follows similar lines to that adopted for the acquired disease, though sometimes of course, additional local measures are required. But, naturally, it is impossible to rebuild a congenital syphilitic into a normal human being. His danger as a source of infection (which is, incidentally, very slight) is destroyed – or at any rate, brought down to the level of any other person treated for syphilis. Such conditions as the Clutton's joints are markedly improved, and there is some restoration of normal sight, especially when penicillin is employed. But nothing can abolish such stigmata as Hutchinson's teeth or the saddle nose. When I say 'nothing', I mean nothing in the way of ordinary treatment such as a VD clinic can provide. It would be possible, of course – and in Harold's case I advised it as necessary – for the sufferer to have all his teeth recapped or extracted and replaced by a denture. Saddle nose can be remedied and fairly well reconstructed by plastic surgery in certain selected cases, though in many the surgeon prefers not to operate when there is a history of congenital or tertiary syphilis – which are, except in the method of infection, similar to all intents and purposes.

What can be done by modern treatment is of the utmost value, however, and once again penicillin has proved a step forward, particularly in relieving the 'rheumatic' conditions. But the chief benefit of treatment is that it arrests entirely the further progress of the disease. So here the basic rule applies as elsewhere in the treatment of venereal diseases generally, the sooner treatment is taken, the better, from the points of view of both immediate gain and future welfare. For this reason no one responsible for the care of infants should fail to refer to a specialist the very slightest suspicion of a syphilitic symptom in their charges. As I have already pointed out, the undoubted decrease in the number of cases of congenital syphilis is due in very large measure to the higher standard of child care now observed, and, no less, to the fact that the welfare service is available today to every mother irrespective of her income or social standing.

Harold's case was in so many ways remarkably typical a one of congenital syphilis that I have used him so far as a model on which to point out some of the characteristic features of the disease. Yet there was a personal side to it as well – and this, as always, proved in many ways the most perplexing and absorbing aspect. Before passing on to it, however, I do not think it can be too strongly or too often emphasized that not every case of congenital syphilis reveals the features I have enumerated in Harold's. On the contrary, the disease takes very many forms, and, as with tertiary acquired syphilis, it is so protean and imitates so many other conditions that often it passes unrecognized for what it is. This is something that doctors in general practice, no less than the ordinary public, should always bear in mind.

Harold was not by any means a co-operative patient so far as tracing the history of his case was concerned. At first, he asserted flatly that he could throw no light at all upon the case. He was at pains to point out that he could not have acquired venereal disease, since, as he put it, he 'had never been interested in women'. I replied that there was no suspicion of acquired syphilis, and that his whole condition pointed conclusively to its congenital origin. This – such is the state of the public mind in these matters – seemed to relieve him greatly. On the other hand, by lifting from his shoulders what he thought was a burden of unjustified moral suspicion, it also tended to make him take an indifferent attitude as though tracing the origin of the disease was no concern of his.

Little by little, however, he came to give me some information. I inquired if his parents were still alive.

'Yes', he replied. 'That is to say, my father is. I can barely remember my mother. She died when I was quite a kid – I must have been about five or six at the time. Anyway it's a heck of a time ago. As for dad, he's just plain bats, and always has been, more or less, so you're not likely to get much sense out of him.'

'Tell me about your father,' I urged. I was anxious for every little piece of information, no matter how trivial or irrelevant it might appear.

He told me. His father, an ordinary member of the middle class, had been a bit of a rolling stone, unable to settle for long at anything. He had been first a clerk and then a salesman and finally had opened a small business of his own. He had managed to develop this and it seemed to have been the most successful of his various experiments in living – perhaps because shortly after he commenced it he married, and his wife had no doubt seen to it that he did not let his attention wander too freely. On the death of his wife, he inherited from her a not insignificant sum of money – Harold did not know what its capital value was – but at any rate it was large enough to bring in sufficient to live on modestly. Harold's father – his name was Thomas – saw in it release from the drudgery of work and an opportunity for indulging his roving spirit. He sold his business and, having arranged for small Harold to live with some relatives, who took little interest in him – he made several trips abroad.

'I came to look on my uncle and aunt more as my parents than dad,' said Harold, who, having overcome his initial reluctance to talk had now swung to the opposite extreme and seemed eager to take the whole day in recollecting his life story. 'I didn't see much of him, and when he did turn up, he was practically a stranger. I don't think he cared much about me anyway. If I happened to be at school when he returned to this country from one of his trips, he never took the trouble to come down and see me.'

'You were at boarding school?' I asked. This seemed an important point. Whatever school it was it could not have a very efficient medical officer, else surely the development of those teeth would have been noticed.

'Yes – of a sort,' he replied grimly. 'You know the old idea, doctor – any school you pay for is better than going to a council school. I only wish I had gone to a council school. It was just one of those small private affairs with three overworked masters to look after about a hundred of us.'

'I think I know what you mean,' I commented. 'Weren't you ever medically examined or anything like that?'

'Only if we were ill,' he replied. 'If there wasn't anything wrong in the sense of it being necessary for us to go to bed, all that happened was that the Head Master wrote to our parents and suggested we should see our own doctor during the holidays. I suppose,' he added bitterly, 'you think my condition should have been noticed before?'

'The thought did cross my mind, though I don't know if there was anything to detect,' I returned. 'That's where you can help me. All the same I think your teeth should have been noticed. Your mouth's in a terrible state, you know. No,' I added quickly, 'I don't mean the Hutchinson's teeth – I'm talking about its general state.'

'Oh, I've never had good teeth,' he answered casually.

'No, I don't suppose you have,' I observed. 'When did you first notice anything out of the way?'

'You mean as regards this business?' he rejoined. 'Well,' he went on, as I nodded affirmatively, 'I don't know. I never suspected anything of the kind until the Army MO packed me off to see you – and even then I didn't believe it. I know how scared they are of VD and I thought perhaps he was the sort of man that's likely to see it anywhere, even where it did not exist ...'

'But your knees for example – you must have noticed those?' I asked.

'I suppose I did,' he replied. 'But not very much. I did have some odd pains and aches about me for some time – since, now when would it be? Oh, soon after I left school.'

'After you left school?' I asked. 'What age was that?'

'Oh, I left early. I was just over fifteen when I turned out and got a job as a warehouse clerk.'

'I see. Then sometime between fifteen and now – that's in the past three years, roughly – you've been suffering from pains and discomfort in the joints. Now we're getting on a bit. And the swellings at the knees? What about them?'

'I can't really say when,' he answered. 'Maybe a year ago – not more. After those aches and pains, you see, I just took it that I was a rheumaticky sort of chap and that the swellings were all part of it.'

'You didn't see a doctor about them?'

He shook his head. 'No,' he replied. 'I didn't think it worth while. They didn't hurt. I'm not one to go chasing after doctors for every little thing.'

'I see. What about your sight? Didn't you do anything about that? I should have thought that that would have been important to you if you were a clerk.'

'As a matter of fact, I did think of doing something about it. That didn't turn up till a few months ago. I noticed my right eye was getting a bit bloodshot and that I couldn't see so well, especially in bright light, but I decided to put it off. You see, I knew I'd be getting my call up soon, and I thought the Army people would find out if there was anything wrong and see about it. I didn't see why I should spend good money on glasses when I could get 'em free a little later.'

I made no comment on this, which seemed like putting money values before health or even comfort – though I know that is by no means an uncommon attitude.

'Headaches – what about them?' I went on.

'They were really grim at times – and my eyes used to water so much that I looked as though I had been crying,' he returned. 'But it all cleared up pretty quickly. The left eye sort of repeated the performance and then I just found I couldn't read so well and couldn't stand bright lights. I thought it was just some sort of cold and let it go at that.'

'H'm!' I grunted. This casualness struck me as almost criminally negligent; it does so every time I meet it, which is often, for it is so powerful a reminder of ignorance. But perhaps I am a little too hard on the general public in this respect. Everything he told me was extremely significant – to me; but then I have studied the venereal diseases for a good many years. It is a bad habit of the specialist to imagine that everything which is important to him should be equally so to other people. After all, why should a young man who obviously had not the slightest cause to suspect he had syphilis, interpret every headache or disordered vision as a venereal symptom?

So far, then, I had established one or two useful facts. Harold was a case of quite late congenital syphilis in which the premonitory symptoms had been, so far as could be judged, almost entirely absent. It is probable – almost certain – that abnormalities of the teeth might have been noticed fairly early, but even so they might have escaped attention. Though I pressed him, he could give no account of any rashes or skin eruptions, and the absence of any of the stigmata that these conditions cause bore him out. One of the most common of these signs is rhagades – the skin becomes fissured and crinkled round the mouth and nose. His face was quite innocent of these marks.

'No suggestion was ever made to you by your father that he and your mother had had syphilis?' I asked.

He shook his head. 'No. I can't imagine Dad talking about it anyway. He never went into anything of that sort with me.'

'No, I suppose not,' I murmured, thinking of the number of cases of congenital syphilis in later life that might have been avoided if only parents had the courage to do their duty and warn their children of the facts and the possible lurking danger to them. 'Is he in England now? I mean your father?'

Harold nodded. 'Yes.'

'Have you seen him just lately?'

'Matter of fact, I have,' he answered as though he was making a somewhat surprising statement. 'I've thought it better to keep in touch with him lately.'

'Oh? Why is that?'

'I think the old boy's breaking up,' he replied with a shrug. 'Anyway he's been acting a little strange lately. Getting absent-minded and doesn't seem able to look after himself as he used to.'

'Breaking up?' I repeated. 'But surely he can't be such a very old man?'

'Well, I suppose he's not that old,' Harold returned. 'I suppose he must be round about fifty. I believe he was about thirty when I was born.'

'D'you think he'd see me and talk to me?' I asked. 'I'm anxious to get to the bottom of this business. You see,' I went on, knowing that he might suspect me of 'snooping', 'the more we can learn about the background of these cases, the better it makes things for others.'

'Scientific investigation,' he commented with slight scorn. 'I see. I don't suppose he'd refuse to see you, though whether you'd be able to get anything out of him I don't know. Sometimes it seems he can't remember a single thing.'

'Well, I can try, unless you feel very strongly that I should not,' I remarked.

'I don't mind. I'm more interested in what happens to me now.' In the circumstances that was not an unnatural attitude. His father had done little enough for him – had, in fact, virtually disowned him, if his story was to be believed. He had no particular reason to concern himself unduly with his father's welfare.

'Suppose you think I'm callous,' he remarked shortly. 'Well, I expect I am, but can you blame me – especially after what I know now? What is it you're after? You want to stop him spreading infection, is that it?'

'I wouldn't go as far as that,' I replied, smiling slightly at his aggressiveness. 'You're running ahead a bit too fast. In the first place, I've no evidence to show that your father either has or has had syphilis. Obviously your mother did, else you wouldn't have congenital syphilis, but we don't know that she contracted it from your father. I'm not casting any aspersions on your mother; I'm only stating scientific facts. Then again, even if he did have syphilis, he may have been treated successfully. And finally taking the blackest view and saying that he had syphilis when you were born and has had it untreated ever since, he wouldn't be a very active source of infection. In fact, the chances are that he wouldn't be infectious at all by now.'

Harold stared at me in surprise. 'But I thought ...' he began.

'You thought,' I said, 'that if a man has syphilis and doesn't have it treated he goes on being a danger to others all his life.

That's a widespread popular fallacy. The chief danger is to himself. In the tertiary stage, the disease is non-infectious to all intents and purposes, though there may be periods of relapse when the case may become actively infectious for a short time. But, of course you know what untreated syphilis may lead to, don't you?'

'You go mad, don't you?'

I nodded. 'Yes. And sometimes in very unpleasant ways. Mind and body disintegrate to put it rather crudely. Luckily, I think we've saved you from that danger.'

'Me?' he exclaimed. 'But surely ...'

'I should say that quite a high proportion of cases of GPI today arise out of untreated congenital syphilis, just because the victims – like you – don't realize that their ills are due to syphilis and the non-specialist doctor is also apt to confuse them with other conditions – or again for the reason that there's nothing in the patient's history to suggest acquired syphilis.' I tapped my desk to emphasize the points. 'Don't you admit that but for your Army medical, you'd never have come here or suspected your condition until, perhaps, you'd gone so far that you had to consult a doctor – and then it might have been much too late?'

'Yes, I suppose so,' he said very slowly. After a pause he added, 'I'm all right now – or I shall be, I suppose?'

'Provided you come here regularly for tests to guard against a relapse and to make sure that our treatment's been effective, you won't have much to trouble about,' I replied. 'You're going to have all your teeth out anyway, and you may, if you want to, find a plastic surgeon who'll be ready to correct the slight deformity of your nose. I can pass you on to the other departments of this Clinic for all that. But the first thing is to make certain I've been successful in my job, and I can only do that if you come here regularly for examinations for the next two years. If you move, I can give you a letter to your nearest clinic.'

'I see.' He still seemed slightly appalled by the vision of what he had escaped. I had not put it to him so strongly before. After another thoughtful pause, he looked at me rather shyly and put a question. 'Suppose – suppose,' he said hesitatingly, 'suppose I want to get married later on?'

'You want the blunt truth about that now?' I asked. 'I'm glad you put that question. I should have had to raise it later.'

'I'd rather know now,' he replied, turning his eyes to the floor as though expecting to hear something unpleasant.

'Then this is the position as I see it,' I answered. 'First of all you mustn't have any thought of marriage before your two years tests are finished and they've been negative the whole time.'

'Yes,' he said quietly.

'And then,' I continued, 'my advice is that you shouldn't consider marriage for at least another two years. Furthermore,' I added quickly, seeing that he was about to interrupt me, 'I insist, in fairness to your future wife, that you should come here or go to some other clinic and ask for an examination whenever you should decide to get married, however far it may be in the future.'

'It sounds pretty awful,' he commented.

'It does – all the more so because you're an entirely innocent victim,' I rejoined. 'And even that's not quite all.'

'What else is there?' he asked. 'Surely if I leave it four years there's nothing else to fear?'

'The only thing you can say about syphilis is that once you've given a home to the spirochaete you can never be absolutely certain that you've entirely got rid of it. At least, that is the present position, though the evidence mounts up that the antibiotic drugs are modifying the position very hopefully. Well then,' I went on, 'my advice would be that you should be honest with whoever you want to marry. Tell her the facts – you've nothing to be ashamed of, you know. Get her to admit that almost improbable but not entirely impossible risk and agree that, if she is ever going to have a child, she will submit herself to examination and treatment, as a precaution.'

'How ghastly!' he exclaimed feelingly.

'No, not quite as bad as that, if you take a rational view of it,' I said. 'It's no more than a measuré of common prudence. You wouldn't want a child of yours to repeat your own terrible experience, would you?'

He shook his head firmly.

'Very well, then. Nor, I think, would you want to undergo the torture of having that vague suspicion at the back of your mind and having to keep it there because you'd never had the courage to tell your wife.'

'No, I suppose not,' he said, rather dully.

'And after all what is there in it?' I asked. 'There's nothing very unpleasant about penicillin treatment, as you know. It's quick and the patient isn't confined to hospital for very long – a day or two, in fact. So what it comes down to is that you'll have to be honest if you intend to marry – that's the first essential, and if your wife is the right person she'll honour you for it, depend on it. And secondly, you'll have to take the reasonable view and look on this precautionary treatment as what it is – in exactly the same class as vaccination. The chances of your getting smallpox under modern conditions are small, but the wise person doesn't refuse vaccination on that account, does he? Or innoculation against other diseases either, if he knows they're effective. Nor does anyone think any the less of him for having these precautions and protection.'

'No, I suppose not.' He looked very thoughtful. I think I was putting an entirely new viewpoint of venereal disease to him, and I could imagine that it had come as rather a shock to him. But I felt, too, that once the first shock of novelty had passed, he would see the sound common-sense of the attitude. I am only too glad to testify that modern young people are receptive to right thinking about venereal diseases if the proper picture is presented to them.

'But don't brood on it,' I resumed. 'There's plenty of time, and you're still a little upset about the whole business, so you can't think too clearly about it all. You're young. Even if you wait that four or so years, you'll still be only twenty-two, and that's far from being too old to think about marriage – many people would say it was still too young.' I smiled. 'And now I'm going to ask you a great favour.'

'What is it?' he asked. 'If there's anything I can do for you, doctor, I'd be really glad to do it. I don't mind confessing now I hated you at first – but I suppose it's not unusual to hate people who tell you the truth.' He smiled rather wryly. 'You've been a good friend to me, I can see that now.'

'I hope so,' I said. 'And I hope you'll always look on me as a friend to help you if you need me – though naturally I hope the need won't be professional. I'll only say that later on if the question should arise in a practical way, I'd be only too glad to discuss the marriage problem with you. But about my favour.'

'Yes – please tell me.'

'I want you,' I said seriously, 'to arrange for me to see your father. You've said one or two things to suggest that it would be very wise to let me see him.'

He opened his eyes. 'You don't mean ...?'

I nodded. 'I'm afraid so. It may be only my suspicious mind, but I think it better for everyone concerned for me to see him as soon as possible. I think I may have a chance to save another tragedy in your family. I only hope it won't be too late.'

'GPI, I suppose,' he said in a flat voice.

'I don't know. I can only say that for a man of fifty to be losing his mind after having had a syphilitic child eighteen years before is suspicious.'

He rose. 'All right, doctor,' he said. 'I'll fix it as soon as possible. I don't know what I'll tell him, but I'll find a way.'

He shook my hand and left me.

That was the son, with the father as a vaguely menacing background. With Harold I had been as successful as I could have hoped, not least because I believed I had swung his mind round to a rational approach to the disaster so narrowly averted in his life and its still threatening consequences and implications. Whether one day I should be able to say the same of the father, I did not know. Perhaps my fears were ill-founded and my services would not be needed. It was a chance – but no more.

Case 8

FATHER AND SON

Harold's attitude towards my desire to see his father was rather curious. My impression was that, personally, he would not care if his father was suffering the torments of the damned; in fact I do not know if he would have regarded such a punishment as too savage but would have been rather pleased about it.

For that reason, I half expected that he would try to evade the fulfilment of his promise to arrange an interview for me. In this, I was mistaken. There was another force at work in Harold – gratitude for what I had done for him. He thanked me again and again at almost every one of the visits he paid to me, but there was nothing gushing or formal about his expressions; they were simple, sincere, and in dead earnest. I pointed out to him that I had done little or nothing to deserve all this, for any competent VD specialist working in a modern clinic would have secured exactly the same results, treated him as regards the important psychological approach in a precisely similar way, and, in the end, told him the same unpleasant hard truths about his future conduct. He would have none of it. That is often the way with patients – a survival, I suppose, of the days when medicine was more an empirical art than an exact science, and when so much depended upon (shall I confess it? For it still applies to quite a few branches of medicine) the personal factor and the lucky guess rather than on the application of the results of research.

For this reason, he was anxious to help me to achieve something I obviously desired. It was at the third interview after that at which he undertook to make arrangements, that he brought up the subject in a practical way.

'About Dad, doctor,' he said, when our formal business of

the day was concluded. 'I've been thinking about it, and I think the best thing I can do is to take you down to see him without any preliminaries. I've an idea he would refuse point blank if I wrote to him or went to see him to ask him about it, and my going would put him wise to what was in the wind. He's always hated anything that merely sniffs of interference with his affairs. I wish there was a better way, but I just can't think one up. What worries me is that it may be wasting your time – he might be out when we turned up or even chuck us out.'

'That's a risk we must take, and I don't mind doing so,' I replied. 'I do think it important that he should be examined by a doctor, and in all circumstances I rather feel that it should be my job. On the other hand, if you think he could be more easily induced to see another doctor, I'd be quite willing, of course, to stand out of the way. The point is that I do think it urgent that someone should examine him.'

He shot a curiously penetrating glance at me. In some ways he had changed a good deal since he had first come to see me, and markedly for the better. Now, he was more mature, better able to make up his own mind – in fact he had turned very rapidly from the boy into the man. But he did not comment on what I said, beyond saying that if a doctor was going to see his father, I must be that doctor.

So it was arranged. He was to call at the Clinic the following Monday soon after lunch, and I was to take him down with me in the car. Thomas, Harold's father, lived in a suburb a few miles north of the Clinic. I warned Harold that he had better telephone me on the Monday morning to make sure that I could fulfil the engagement, for there was always a chance, as with every doctor in practice, that something vitally urgent might be occupying my attention.

Nothing turned up, however, and at half-past-two on the day, he and I set out on the journey. Apart from anything else, I was not sorry to get away from the Clinic for a little while, especially as I had had a case which had tied me to the place over the entire weekend.

'That's the place,' said Harold suddenly, as we drove slowly along a side road. 'The cottage by itself there.'

I was pleasantly surprised. The house looked like a relic of the days when this district had been rural and had not been engulfed in the flood of bricks that had flowed out from the town. It looked clean, comfortable, and homely.

'Now,' said Harold, as I stopped the car, 'we'll see what's going to happen. Mrs Butters is a good landlady maybe, but she does not like me. She thinks I'm an unnatural son who doesn't do his duty because I don't spend all my spare time with the old man. You know what these old people are.'

I nodded, but made no observation. He knocked at the door – the brass knocker gleamed brightly – and he braced himself a little, I thought, when the door began to open. Mrs Butters, a pleasant-looking old lady with well brushed, sparse grey hair done in a little knot at the back of her head, stared at him – and I prepared for the chilly reception he had forecast. But he was wrong. As soon as she recognized him, her face beamed with relief.

'Oh, Mr Harold,' she exclaimed, 'I'm so glad you've come! I'd been half inclined to write to you, but I didn't want to seem to be pushing myself into your business. Your father's not been very well lately, and I'm rather worried about him.'

'I'm sorry, Mrs Butters,' said Harold. 'What's the matter?'

She glanced inquiringly at me as though wondering whether she could speak freely.

Harold interpreted the glance. 'Oh, this is a friend of mine, Mrs Butters. He's a doctor – Dr Jonathan Miles, of the Maynard Clinic. You can say what you like in front of him. In fact, he's come down with me specially to see Dad.'

She looked at me with the faintest suspicion of a little bob of respect. 'I'm very pleased to meet you, sir,' she said. 'That's one of the things I've been thinking about – sending for a doctor. I'm glad you've come, sir – you're very welcome.' Her expression changed to dismay. 'But what on earth am I thinking of, keeping you here talking at the door. Oh, please do forgive me, sir! Come in – come in.'

She led the way into a trim little parlour that held, among a miscellaneous collection of old-fashioned furniture, a stuffed owl in a glass case, which looked down from the mantelpiece with the air of a presiding deity.

'Now tell me, Mrs Butters,' I said when she had offered us tea, which we refused, 'what is the matter with Harold's father?'

She looked at me seriously. 'I don't rightly know, sir,' she replied earnestly. 'It's just that he's so odd. When he first come here – let me see, that would be about fifteen years ago – how time flies! Yes, sir, when he first come here, he was always so spruce and active and looked after himself so well. He told me he'd been abroad a lot and got used to looking after himself. But I couldn't let him darn his socks, sir, like he wanted to – it isn't right and proper for a man to use a needle.'

'No, Mrs Butters,' I interposed. 'But you were telling us that he was odd – that was the word.'

'Yes, sir, but it's him being so tidy in the past that makes it so very funny now. You see, there are times when he just won't take any care of himself at all. He won't even wash his hands, sir, or shave. And the mess he makes when he has a meal, you'd never believe! He gets it all over himself, sir, if you don't mind me telling you these things and he doesn't so much as trouble to wipe it off.'

The doubts I had entertained that I might be on a wild-goose chase grew suddenly less. Mrs Butter's news was rather more than disquieting, to say the least.

'How is he today?' I asked.

She shook her head in puzzlement. 'Oh, he's quite all right today, sir,' she replied in a voice of surprise. 'That's the funny thing about it all – one day he's as right as a trivet and the next he hardly seems to be in his right mind. Oh, I'm sorry I said it like that, Mr Harold,' she added quickly, but Harold reassured her with a smile.

'I see,' I said. 'Well, perhaps we shall know more about it when we've talked to him.' I did not wish to ask any more questions; I had an impression that Mrs Butters might be just a little too ready to oblige and agree to the vaguest suggestion I might make.

'When can we go up?'

'Straightaway, sir,' she replied. 'I'll show the way. Oh, of course, there's no need,' she added. 'You know, don't you, Mr Harold?'

Harold nodded. 'Don't you trouble, Mrs Butters,' he said. 'In any event I think it better we shouldn't be formally announced. He's often not ready to see me and he might take great offence at having two visitors.'

'Yes, Mr Harold,' commented Mrs Butters, nodding sagely. 'There's a lot of truth in that. He needs a mort of handling.'

I followed Harold up the narrow, creaking staircase, which, like everything else in the house, no matter how aged it might be, was spotlessly clean. The paintwork at the edges of the narrow strip of well-brushed stair-carpet was as white as the day it had been applied. Harold paused for a moment at the head of the stairs and then advanced towards a door on his right, on which he tapped three times.

'Yes?' said a voice from within. 'Who is it? Come in.'

Harold signed me to follow and entered the room.

'Why, Harold!' exclaimed Thomas. 'Come to see me at last, have you? And about time, too. Why don't you answer my letters?'

Harold opened his eyes wide. 'Letters, Dad? I've never had any.'

'Oh!' Thomas was obviously about to make some cutting remark, when he caught sight of me in the shadow of the doorway. 'Hullo, who's this?' he demanded in a not very friendly way.

'A friend of mine,' answered Harold. 'Jonathan Miles. He kindly brought me down in his car.'

We had agreed, to start with, I should not be introduced as a doctor, though I determined to correct any misconceptions that concealed identity might produce at the earliest possible moment.

'Well, come in,' he grunted, looking at me. 'Shut the door after you. As you're here you may as well stay.'

It was not a very encouraging welcome, and the accompanying look of suspicion did not belie the words. I prepared myself for a difficult interview. On the way in the car, Harold and I had come to an agreement that he should do most of the talking to start with in order to feel the way gradually.

Harold dropped into a nearby chair and waved me to

another. I took a quick look around. The room was unexceptional, indeed it was a very nice bed-sitting-room, spacious, comfortably furnished, and, of course, beautifully kept. I was more interested in the occupant than in the environment, however, though sometimes the latter can be very informative. Thomas was easily recognizable as Harold's father, for the family resemblance was most marked. He looked, however, old for his years – assuming Harold's estimate of his age, about fifty, to be correct, and his expression was one of bad temper and impatience. As he sat, with his back to the light by the side of the fireplace, it was not easy to see more, especially as I was making my inspection as surreptitiously as possible.

'How are you feeling, Dad?' asked Harold.

It was an innocent enough question, and quite a natural one in any circumstances, but Thomas bridled at once and looked with deep suspicion at his son.

'What made you ask that?' he demanded roughly. 'The old girl been talking to you?'

'What do you mean, Dad?' fenced Harold. 'Haven't you been well lately?'

'I'm all right,' he replied brusquely. 'Nothing the matter with me. Why should there be? But that old girl seems to think I'm an invalid and need looking after. Even suggested I ought to see a doctor. Why? Simply because sometimes I feel a bit lazy and don't wash or shave for a day. Why shouldn't I? My own business entirely. Besides, I'm starting to get on, you know, and it's natural I ought to feel like relaxing. Scrub – scrub – scrub – that woman never stops and I suppose she'd like to start on me as well. She can keep it.'

'You're not so old, Dad,' said Harold, who, for all his youth, seemed to me to be handling the situation very well.

'Maybe, but fifty-one is old enough for me. I've led a pretty active life and I expect I've worn myself out early – that's about it. The only thing the matter with me is that I feel ruddy tired nowadays. Satisfied? Any more questions?'

I had listened to all this with great intentness. The suggestion that he was ill had touched him on a sore spot and his indignation was as much defence-by-attack as anything else. For one moment, when he had so tersely summed up Mrs Butters as 'scrub – scrub – scrub' I had wondered whether she had exaggerated; and then, as he had shifted a little in his chair, and I had seen the impressive (and depressing) array of food and saliva stains on his coat, the doubt instantly disappeared.

Harold glanced quickly at me. Clearly he felt, as I did, that we should get nowhere along these lines, and I decided to intervene.

'It was a pleasure for me to bring Harold down here,' I said, apparently to make conversation, 'and I welcome the chance because I've been wanting to speak to you for some time.'

He turned towards me. I was sitting a little behind him, and as he swivelled he came more into the light so that I was able to see him more clearly. I had chosen my position well.

'Oh, and what does all this mean?' he demanded.

'I am a doctor,' I replied, and his expression grew grim. 'For some time past I have been treating Harold for a certain condition, and I should like to talk it over with you.'

'Well?'

'Your son has been suffering from congenital syphilis,' I said calmly.

He half rose from his chair in indignation. 'What's that to do with me?' he shouted. 'He's old enough to look after himself, and if he goes playing the bloody fool, that's his look out. It's no concern of mine. In any event I thought you doctors treated all cases like that in complete secrecy.'

'I think you misheard me,' I returned, still keeping calm. 'I said congenital syphilis – and that does concern you closely.'

'How he got it is of no interest to me.'

'I don't think you quite understand,' I persisted. 'Harold was infected with syphilis before he was born, but, as so often happens, it did not appear in a recognizable form till just recently. It is my duty to investigate the history of all such cases, and that's why I've come to you.'

'I know better than that,' he retorted slyly. 'Even if you're right it's no business of mine. He got it from his mother, and she is dead.'

I insisted. I told him that what he said was quite correct,

but that if she was syphilitic and had not been treated, the odds-on chances were that he himself had been syphilitic, too. And in any case, what I wanted was information for the purposes of scientific study as I was a specialist in venereal diseases.

'I know nothing about it,' he said obstinately.

He was still facing towards me with the light on his face. I drew out my cigarette and a box of matches, though I usually use a lighter. Slowly I lit a cigarette and I let the match burn, holding it high as though I was lost in thought. It was only a little distance from his eyes, but he did not even blink. Then, suddenly he turned his head away.

'You silly fool!' he said. 'Light like that hurts my eyes. Age again I suppose.'

To me it was a sign not without significance, especially when added to the other things I had noticed while I had been talking to him. First of all there had been the marked irregularity of the pupils of the eyes, one being much larger than the other; and when I had held out that lighted match there had been an appreciable pause before they had begun slowly and reluctantly to adapt themselves to the change in light intensity; normal pupils would have contracted quite rapidly under such conditions. Then again his facial muscles, particularly round the mouth, had been in a constant state of fine tremor – almost unnoticeable to the untrained eye but quite characteristic in its own way. On the right temple was a patch of faint discoloration that many would have passed off as the remains of a fairly old bruise, but the skin on it was atrophic – that is to say it was degenerate, structureless skin – and it seemed to me a tell-tale indication of a healed tertiary syphilitic lesion – a syphilide, as it is termed.

My mind was already made up. Here, I felt, was a case of very long-established tertiary syphilis – and it was on the verge of disaster. The muscle tremor and the sluggishness of the eye reactions were highly suspicious, taken in conjunction with the indications Mrs Butters had given us of mental deterioration. Thomas must, by hook or by crook, be removed to the Clinic for examination and possible treatment.

I had advanced so far and was considering the next step,

while Harold gave me an anxious glance, when a remarkable thing happened. It was almost as if Thomas, sitting in his chair, had assumed another personality. Suddenly, without a word, he grew completely listless to the point of seeming ignorant of our presence. He passed his hand, with the air of a man utterly worn out, over his brow. I watched him closely, waiting before I took any active part in the situation.

'My head – oh, these terrible headaches!' he groaned.

It was not so much the description of the symptom that interested me though it was quite important in its way, as the voice in which the words were spoken. It was slurred, indistinct, as though he had difficulty in controlling his tongue.

'Tell me more about them,' I said softly.

He took no notice. I repeated the question. At the third attempt he made a reluctant movement with his head towards me.

'Eh?' he drawled. 'What?'

The fourth repetition of the question sank in.

'My head,' he said slowly and with difficulty. 'Comes on suddenly like this.'

I did not press him, but, rising I made a sign for Harold to follow me out of the room. On the landing I put my suspicions strongly to him.

'Your father is in a very dangerous state,' I said. 'Dangerous, I mean, for himself, not that he might get violent in any way. He carries many of the signs that suggest advanced tertiary syphilis to me, though, of course, I can't be sure without a proper examination, and more than that he looks to me as though he's already got general paresis – GPI.'

'God!' exclaimed Harold. 'What's to be done?'

'We must get him to the Clinic at the earliest possible moment and see if my suspicions are confirmed or dismissed. But even if it's not what I think it is, he still needs treatment.'

'But there's nothing you can do for GPI, is there?' asked Harold. 'I mean, nothing except shut him up in an asylum?'

'There's always hope, though I don't disguise the fact that the outlook is never very rosy in such cases,' I replied. 'But we can do a lot today, you know, and there's no need to give way to despair. Even in the worse cases, it's usually possible to effect some sort of improvement, and in more favourable circumstances it's more than likely there'd be a complete cure. But the thing today is to act promptly. Do you agree? Have I your permission to take him to the Clinic? The responsibility rests with you, for I feel that he is not capable himself of making a rational decision.'

'Of course,' replied Harold with a note of surprise. 'Why on earth should you ask?'

'A matter of form,' I returned with a smile. 'One has to do these things.'

I went back to the bed-sitting-room to find Thomas is practically the same position as I had left him. This was not a very encouraging state of affairs from the general point of view, but it was a helpful condition in view of what I had to do. He was not likely to make any resistance to his removal. In fact, when we got his things together and helped him down to the car – I had decided not to call an ambulance – he seemed to take no interest at all in the proceedings. An hour earlier, in his mood of aggressive irrascibility, he might even have resorted to physical violence in resisting an interference with his affairs. These sudden changes of mood and temper are characteristic of general paresis, but they are by no means conclusive. Purely mental disorders may produce them, as, for example, dementia praecox.

On arrival at the Clinic, to which I had telephoned en route so as to have a bed ready for him, I decided to leave him overnight and to carry out my examination in the morning. The examination has to be extremely thorough, for, as I have just said, many of the signs and symptoms of GPI are identical with those of purely psychotic states, and even the physical manifestations may be due to non-syphilitic causes. A very careful differentiation of every aspect has to be made, therefore, but most important of all are the tests of the cerebro-spinal fluid, specimens of which are withdrawn by the technique of lumbar puncture. General paresis and other distressing states, among them locomotor ataxia or tabes dorsalis, are due to the invasion of the central nervous system by the spirochaetal infection. These parts of the human body are the last to surrender their defences to the invading toxins; before they do so, the whole body has been sapped and undermined, and there is usually ample evidence of the progress distributed throughout the whole body.

When the time came, I discovered what almost was conclusive clinical evidence of long-standing untreated syphilis in Thomas. The disease was still active in him to some extent, no doubt reappearing again after a period of apparent quiescence. One of the grossest signs was the existence, on the abdominal surface, of a patch of syphilides or gummata – the typical tertiary lesion, which showed advanced ulceration. Many bones and joints were involved, and there was also evidence of infection of some of the glands and blood vessels. On his right hand, one of the nails had peeled right off, while the nails of the left hand showed another and more repulsive type of infection known as paronychia, which results in purulent swellings at the base of the nails. I had no doubt that the 'bruise' mark I had observed on his forehead was the stigma left by an earlier gummatous infection.

Altogether, I would have been justified in diagnosing tertiary syphilis on the clinical evidence alone. It was astonishing to me that any man could have allowed himself not merely to advance to such a state but also to accept it without treatment of any kind. Yet even with all these indications in front of me, I could not say with perfect scientific certainty that this was indeed tertiary syphilis. The last and conclusive proof lay with the tests on the cerebro-spinal fluid.

Several tests were made on this fluid, but the most important and crucial one is the Wassermann reaction. Though I felt that this could not be but positive, I had to await the report of the serologist before initiating any sort of treatment. By the next day, I should know.

Meanwhile, Thomas was kept quiet. He remained for the remainder of the day in a state of semi-stupor. If he had behaved in his lodgings as he did in the private ward in which he had been placed, I do not wonder that Mrs Butters was worried about him; his habits would have shocked many a person far less scrupulous on matters of cleanliness than she was. A well trained dog or cat – or even a pig – would have been a far more pleasant and hygienic companion.

Of course, the laboratory reports were positive on every head. I was faced with a case of advanced neuro-syphilis – and a few years ago that would have meant a completely hopeless outlook. But today this condition can be treated with quite high hopes of success unless the patient is in a very advanced state of GPI when he presents himself. The accepted method is what is known as fever therapy, which involves inoculating the patient with some form of fever and maintaining him in that condition for a longer or shorter time according to the severity of the case, and repeating it as necessary. Each innoculation is, of course, followed at the desired time by curative measures to dispel the fever combined with high doses of antibiotics.

At various times, many different types of fever have been employed for this treatment, but today the use of inoculations of malaria are practically universal, not only because it gives the most satisfactory results in itself but because the fever itself is readily controlled. The man – Professor Wagner von Yaureck of Vienna University – who introduced this treatment was awarded the Nobel Prize for Medicine.

Fever therapy is, as can be imagined, a fairly drastic form of treatment and it has to be administered with great care. Before inoculation can be attempted, the patient has to be in as sound a condition physically as it is possible to make him. It is difficult and not without risk where old people are concerned, and often the long-standing syphilis which leads up to the onset of general paresis has wrought considerable havoc with the patient's general condition.

So it was with Thomas. His heart and blood vessels had been affected by the disease, and there was also some doubt about his liver. No alternative existed to delaying the application of fever therapy until such time as we had done something to build him up.

This worried Harold to some extent. He had now, rather belatedly and in the face of overt danger, developed a good deal of concern for his father. In a sense, I feel that it was more reaction to his own experience than any sudden upsurging or filial affection. 'There,' he was repeating to himself, 'but for the grace of God, I go.' He could not reconcile my previous insistence on the need for immediate treatment with my present apparent dilatoriness, but when I explained the position to him he appeared to understand.

It was during this period of uneasy intermission that Thomas's condition took a new turn, perfectly in keeping with the state of general paresis. His general mood of depression and lethargy suddenly disappeared and he began to have the famous delusions of grandeur. Sometimes, as is well known, these delusions take the most fantastic forms, the sufferer imagining himself to be some great figure of history or legend. Thomas's delusions, however, took a more practical form; he obviously saw himself as the great organizational genius and administrator. This is not so very uncommon, and it is because the delusions do take this form (and often in the most rational-seeming way) that tertiary syphilitics have shown an amazing power of direction and ability, which suddenly and inexplicably evaporates. I believe myself that if Thomas had been still on his own during these stages, he might have achieved something quite spectacular.

The nurse, entering the ward one morning and expecting to find her patient in bed, was surprised to see him standing, in his dressing-gown, by the window. The Maynard Clinic stands in its own grounds and the view from the window was by no means unattractive. But its practical details did not appeal to the new Thomas.

'I've been watching the traffic,' he observed without preliminaries. 'The arrangements here are quite inefficient. The cars and vans approaching the building have to make a wide detour round that ornamental lake – which itself, I see, is in bad condition. That lake should be bridged. Will you please arrange for the person responsible for buildings and so on to come and see me?'

'Yes,' said the nurse, not unused to this sort of thing. She reported the matter to me, and when I went to visit him later in the morning he mistook me for the Clerk of the Works.

'You've been a long time answering my summons,' he remarked sharply.

'I've been busy,' I replied.

'No doubt. But this is important,' he rejoined. 'However, the time hasn't been wasted. I've been able to draft out a rough scheme for you to work on. Take it away and let me see something based on it tomorrow. I don't want a report. I merely want the details worked out.'

I took his documents away with me. They were interesting from two points of view. The most important from my own standpoint was that they contained further evidence of his condition. The writing was shaky and gave a sense of insecurity; the nerve paralysis was affecting the muscles of his hands and arms. Common words too, were misspelt in the most ridiculous way – which again is typical of general paresis. Thus 'bridge' appeared in two places as 'brij', 'road' as 'rode', and 'white' as 'wite' – to give only three examples from many. On the other hand, some words were left out, making the sense of the whole a little obscure in places. 'The brij be bilt stone desired' was one sentence, showing both misspelling and omissions; it meant, I gathered, that the bridge be built of stone, if desired.

The other interesting point was that an engineer friend of mine to whom I showed the scheme which included some rough drawings not at all badly executed, assured me that it was quite practicable and that the steel bridge he had sketched was technically correct. It was, in fact, a perfectly good plan – provided one wished to spend several tens of thousands of pounds so that visitor's cars and tradesmens' vans could save perhaps forty five seconds on their journey from gates to the Clinic buildings.

Next day his ideas had grown a little more sweeping. He nodded to me shortly as I came in, as a business man of high responsibilities might greet an inferior and employee.

'The scheme will have to be revised,' he said as soon as he saw me. 'The rough one I gave you doesn't go far enough. The approach road must be straightened and widened, and that, of course, will mean a larger bridge. That little wood will have to be moved.'

From his position by the window he pointed out a small beech copse, the pride of the Clinic.

'Of course,' he went on, 'I quite understand that people would object to cutting down those trees. I've worked out a plan to avoid it. All we have to do is to dig a deep, narrow trench right round the wood and then cross cut beneath the roots of the trees. As the excavations proceed, we inject concrete and finally we fill up the surrounding trench. So you've got the whole wood in a concrete tank. With suitable cranes and derricks you can lift up the whole wood, just as it is, and put it down in a more convenient position. It's really a very simple process, don't you see? It has hundreds of applications. I shall bring it up at the next council meeting of the Institution.'

'The Institution?' I queried.

He nodded gravely. 'Yes – the Civil Engineers, of course. Didn't I tell you I had been asked to stand for the Presidency next year? I shall make my new method of shifting woods the subject of my presidential address.'

So that was it. In two days he had risen from a tamperer with the layout of an ancient estate to President Elect of the Institution of Civil Engineers. For some unfathomable reason he was seeing himself as a great engineer. This was the key – for there is always a key to these depressions, a connecting link that is wholly consistent and rational, in the sense of being logical once the premises are granted. And in the next few days, he was planning the most grandiose schemes – tunnelling the Atlantic (or alternatively spanning it by a huge highway supported on floating platforms, an idea he worked out in some details, to the amazement and admiration of my civil engineer friend); cutting a canal wide and deep enough to take ocean-going ships right across Europe and disgorging direct into Suez; making London a vast two decker city with the upper part devoted to aerodromes, parks, and playing grounds, and the lower affording a covered over series of roads and pavements where the townspeople could go about their affairs unconcerned by weather – for the streets were air conditioned and lighted by artificial sunlight. His imagination soared higher and higher; there seemed no end to his fanciful notions; which were all the more remarkable in that all held at least a measure of common sense and detailed planning.

It was an interesting case of systematic delusions, but from the point of view of my proposed treatment for his condition, it was not at all a favourable development. He was far too active in mind and body, too, to accept quietly a regimen that entailed confinement to bed and a diet designed to build up his strength. I could only gamble on the probability that it was but a temporary phase and that soon there would be a reversion to his former depressive state.

I was right in expecting that the chances of a relapse from this exaltation would ensue, but I was wrong in believing that it would be to a state of lethargy. Far from it. About ten days later I was called to his ward by a rather troubled nurse who reported that the patient was 'going off the deep end' in real earnest. I found Thomas sitting up in bed, looking as bed-tempered as I have ever seen a man, and obviously ready to set about any person who dared to cross his path.

'What the hell am I doing here and who are you?' he stormed as soon as I entered the ward.

'I'm the director of this section of the Maynard Clinic,' I replied, thinking it better not to be too precise about my department, 'and you are here because you have been and still are seriously ill.'

'Seriously ill? That be damned. I'm as fit as a fiddle, and I propose to leave this instant. Who sent me here and when?'

'You've been here rather more than a fortnight,' I answered, 'and you are certainly not going to leave. On the contrary, we are just about to commence a new and important phase of your treatment.'

'I'm not ill,' he asserted. 'What is it supposed to be?'

'Can you remember yesterday or the day before?' I asked, evading the issue.

He wrinkled his brow. 'No,' he said slowly at last. 'My memory seems a little muddled. I see. I'm a head case.'

He sank back on the pillow. Now he was concerned with the loss of memory, as he put it. Everything he said and did was, to me, an urgent reminder that treatment could be no longer delayed. And when, the next day, the night nurse told me that he was losing all sense of time and place, I knew that his condition was deteriorating far too rapidly for my liking.

'He keeps asking when his wife's coming to see him,' she remarked. 'It's quite pathetic and rather sweet, really. She never comes, does she?'

'No,' I replied grimly. 'This is a VD clinic not a paranormal research laboratory. She died fourteen or fifteen years ago.'

'Oh!' she said and shot me a significant glance. Her experience of these cases was fairly wide and she knew what his question meant. It is when the time-sense begins to become utterly confused and 'yesterday' comes to mean anything from an hour ago to twenty-five years before – or paradoxically, tomorrow, for that curious inversion has occurred – that one has proof of the serious state of the mental processes. More often the development of the full picture of general paresis is slow and continuous, with only brief interludes of comparative normality. Thomas's case was forging ahead by leaps and bounds. I did not like it and told the nurses so. When Harold came that afternoon, I told him too, and warned him that the outlook was grave.

Obviously treatment could no longer be put off. Thomas was not in the general condition I should have liked him to have been, but a risk had to be taken if all hope of saving something from the wreck was not to be abandoned. That evening I inoculated Thomas with malarial blood. Even now there would be a week or so to wait, for the inoculation period of the strain I had used was seven days, and meanwhile there was little to do but wait.

One cannot make accurate predictions of the behaviour of these patients, and I did not know what to expect. His delusions might return before the fever manifested itself; he might continue to be more or less normal, with a violently expressed resentment to everyone and everything; or he might become lethargic and docile. In the event, it turned out that he developed the last-named condition. It was so marked that I had to keep constant observation to reassure myself that it was really a mental symptom and not a sign of general collapse.

There is no need to go into details of the fever therapy. It is a difficult and anxious method for doctors and nurses alike. But here at least Thomas, though unconsciously so, was most co-operative. He accepted the full course I had decided upon as desirable without showing any untoward developments, and he was comparatively little trouble to his nurses. At the end of it all, I was reasonably well satisfied. He had been prepared for the fever therapy by treatment with iodides and arsenical and bismuth compounds as well as with penicillin, though, in view of his general condition, I had had to use the last named two rather sparingly. Now the main part of this stage was over, a fresh phase began – one more akin to the general treatment of syphilis in its earlier stages. Thomas, still retained in hospital, for it was highly undesirable that he should be allowed anywhere without proper control always at hand, was started now on an intensive course of penicillin and the arsenical compounds. Penicillin gives remarkable results in these cases, so do the other antibiotic drugs when the patient is allergic to penicillin, but the data relating to antibiotic therapy, especially as regards the final outcome, is still too sparse to enable us to rely on it exclusively, though I am more than hopeful of what the final verdict will be. The only safe course, therefore, is to employ penicillin and the other antibiotic drugs more as adjunct to older and more proven treatments than as a complete therapy by itself. It is possible, I believe, without any undue risks, to reduce the other treatments somewhat or even to discard them all together in certain cases, though in Thomas's case I kept them up for the ten weeks established by considerable experience.

It was clear that a great improvement had been worked on him. As he slowly recovered, his mind cleared wonderfully. I did not expect a complete cure. The lesions in some of his bones and joints and the damage done to the heart and liver could never be repaired fully, and there would always be the danger of sudden relapse. GPI is an occult curtain that cannot be swept aside rather than a shadow that can be dispersed by light.

There arose, therefore, the problem of what was to be done with him. He could not be allowed to return to his former apartments and the sole care of Mrs Butters, who, although a thoroughly estimable woman, could not, in human justice, have such a man inflicted upon her; nor was she capable of handling any emergency that might arise. Moreover, it is necessary to carry out examinations, allied to serological tests of the blood and the cerebro-spinal fluid, over an extended period, some times for as long as five years. Some means had to be devised of ensuring that he should submit to these with unfailing regularity.

At last, after consulting with Harold, I arranged for him to be sent for the time being, at any rate, to one of the two homes affiliated to the Maynard Clinic for the reception of chronic cases of various kinds. There he would be in thoroughly competent hands, and I would be able to keep him under the closest observation.

For some months after the conclusion of the active treatment he made steady progress and attained to a clarity of mind and memory I would hardly have thought possible. During this time, he came to realize the seriousness of the condition he had been in, and he grew quite humble and contrite about it. Moreover, he gave me quite a wealth of detail which threw considerable light upon his own case and Harold's as well.

The truth, as it emerged piecemeal in a series of talks with him, was terrible enough. He had always been 'weak with women', to use his own, oft-repeated phrase, and there were moments when he did not care with whom he resorted so long as he was able to satisfy his appetite for them. His marriage was, on his side, one of purely practical politics. He had been wise enough to realize that the life he was leading was a sure short cut to ruin in every sense, and he felt that, if he married, he would be able to work out his salvation. His physical desires could be safely appeased, while, at the same time, the responsibility of a wife would, he believed, sober his behaviour generally and give him something to work for.

For a little while, it worked out as he anticipated, but in the long run his ingrained mode of life reasserted itself. He took to extra-marital adventures, and as a result, he developed syphilis. This was about a year before Harold had been born. He and his wife underwent treatment, but refused to attend for periodical examinations when it was formally concluded. No doubt (as all this happened some time ago when techniques were not so well developed) the cure was not complete and relapse occurred. Thus it was that the seeds of syphilis were implanted in the child, to make their appearance eighteen years later. And also, as he admitted, it was the reason why, in the immediately succeeding years, his wife twice conceived and twice miscarried. Her death, it turned out, was due to haemorrhage after the second of these miscarriages. He decided to go abroad.

'After all this, you still didn't think it essential you should undergo a second course of treatment?' I inquired.

'No,' he answered. 'I was going out East, and I decided there was no point in it. It wouldn't make much difference if I brought a little more with me, and besides I knew myself too well. I knew that even if I got cured before I went, I should only get another dose out there. I was made that way.'

I said nothing. This point of view was impossible to combat.

So it went on. Now he was in England, now abroad. The syphilis did not trouble him much on the whole. He got eruptions from time to time, suffered from pains in the joints, realized that his heart was affected and that his sight was growing progressively worse. But he argued that if he went to a doctor, the only recommendation would be a course of anti-syphilitic treatment, and he regarded that as useless. What was the point of it, when he knew he would only pick up the disease afresh later on? It was just a condition of life that, at first unpleasant, later became commonplace, and he adapted himself to it.

As for Harold, he thought the boy had escaped, as he had seemed so healthy a child, and he could barely believe that he himself was, in truth, responsible for Harold's infection, which showed itself only after so many years.

Much more he told me, but that is the gist of the matter, and it gives a fairly complete statement of most of the facts. There is one other curious sidelight that was revealing as giving a clue to the reason for the form his delusions took. All his life he had dreamed of being a great constructional engineer, but he never did more than work as an unskilled labourer on a dam that was being built at a time when he was in the Middle East. Through his delusions he lived, for a little while, the life and ambitions that had burned so strongly in him.

Thomas was contented in the home for a year, and I began to hope that eventually I would be able to describe him as one of my more spectacular successes. It was not to be. An urgent report came through to me one day, about fourteen months after he had been sent there, saying that he had had a relapse, and delusions had returned. He was brought back to the Clinic, and I saw that he was a hopeless case. It is true that second, third, and even more, applications of fever therapy can be given, but this did not seem possible in this instance. He was too weak. The damaged heart was failing rapidly, and the effect of induced malaria would simply have been to substitute one cause of death for another.

A week after his return to the Clinic, he died. Perhaps it was all for the best. In the most favourable circumstances he could only eke out the remainder of his life in a home, over-shadowed by the thought that his days were numbered – and it would have been no consolation to him that his state was due entirely to his own carelessness and lack of a sense of responsibility to himself and others.

For there can be no denying the facts. He had been responsible for the death of his wife and the stillbirth of two of his children. He had brought into the world a son who had looked catastrophe full in the face and only narrowly averted it. And in the end, he had died of his own stupidity. He took with him to the grave as heavy a burden of misdeeds as any could – though not one of those misdeeds is even vaguely condemned by law. From the grave, too, his shadow still stretches across the life of his son and darkens it, for though Harold's body is cured, his mind has been poisoned by the knowledge that he is not as other men are, and that he cannot enter into the business of love and marriage and home-making without the doubts that, in the end, he may think too heavy a price to pay for the things that other young men claim almost as of right.

Case 9

MAISIE

Cases come to the Clinic by many and devious routes and often patients seem surprised and even outraged at finding themselves suspected of suffering from one of the venereal diseases. In the present state of affairs this is not so very surprising, for people will try anything and everything before they will admit to themselves that they have been subject to this particular type of infection. It is true that nowadays there is much more general recognition of the physical dangers of venereal disease, and it is a very curious commentary on the strength of antiquated attitudes that even intelligent, well-informed patients, with quite a good grasp of the main facts of venereal infections, seem to take the view that 'it can't happen to me'. So, even among these, there is a reluctance to be examined in a VD clinic notwithstanding the appearances of signs and symptoms which, in someone else, they would instantly suspect as being venereal.

But it is not only perverted ignorance or real ignorance or a false sense of security that delays the immediate treatment of patients that is so desirable. There are many people of rational outlook who would not fail to report themselves for examination if they had recognized the slightest sign or entertained the vaguest suspicion. Yet sometimes one finds these to be victims of disease of quite long standing. Why is this? It is because the venereal diseases are so protean in their character. Not only can both the principal ones – gonorrhoea and syphilis – but particularly syphilis – stimulate other conditions so closely that even non-specialist doctors may be deceived; sometimes they are almost completely asymptomatic – that is to say, they show no indications of any significance at all. Since very slight signs in the absence of other suspicious factors, may be overlooked by a doctor, it is not surprising that sufferers themselves with little or no knowledge take no notice of them or are utterly unaware of their presence. It is this which constitutes one of the major problems of the control of venereal disease. Obviously it is impossible to insist on routine, compulsory tests for every member of the adult population, let alone the school population as well, though this is the only course that scientific fact would regard as satisfactory. Nevertheless, even without this drastic and all but impossible measure (except perhaps in a completely totalitarian state), much would be done by a wiser approach to the question.

As I have said, quite intelligent people are sometimes unwitting victims, and ignorance of their condition cannot be set against them as a crime or even a misdemeanour, for there is no doubt that if they had had any suspicion they would, as wise people, have been properly examined. They come to the Clinic as a last, desperate resort on the advice of their own doctor, who, all too often, regards the step as a wild, outside chance – when all else has failed.

A case of mine comes to mind as I write these words. It had many interesting features and serves well to show how insidiously and obscurely the venereal disease can go to work.

The principal figure is a young woman named Maisie, though, of course, her husband also comes into the picture, for it is very rarely and only in unusual circumstances that one finds only one partner of a marriage to be infected.

Maisie was a young woman in the late twenties. She was not perhaps above the average in good looks, but she was a very admirable specimen of modern womanhood. Her medical history was excellent, containing nothing but the usual children's diseases, and she told me that she very rarely consulted a doctor because she never felt the need of it. Her life had been spent largely in the open air. She was a keen sportswoman and had played with some success in the better lawn tennis tournaments, and she was an expert swimmer. Her physical condition left nothing to be desired. In her outlook, she was practical, balanced, and uninhibited. Presented with this description of her, I should have said that the possibility of her contracting venereal disease was small, and the chances that she would let it develop untreated were remote.

Five years before she came to see me, she had married. Her husband was some twelve years older than herself, a businessman in a good position. They were extremely fond of each other, shared a variety of common interests, and seemed destined for a happy married life. Both were determined to raise a family. It was through that that the first signs of trouble appeared.

The years went by and Maisie failed to conceive. At first they resigned themselves to a fate that they felt would be only temporary. They were still young enough to have a long future before them and time did not matter particularly. But in the end it became obvious that something was wrong with one of them, and since they did not wish to abandon their ambitions without a struggle, they agreed to take advice.

There is a very widespread belief that when a couple fail to have children and there is no obvious reason for their failure, it is the woman who is more likely to be at fault. This view is not perhaps, borne out by medical investigations, which suggests that infertility among men is of fairly high prevalence. This is not a subject to discuss here; the only point is that its acceptance led naturally to Maisie's submitting herself first to a doctor.

A very thorough physical examination was carried out on her, and, of course, nothing wrong was found. She was, as I have already said, a very fine example of fit humanity. Quite rightly, the doctor decided that her low fertility, if it existed, was due to some temporary disturbance. He gave her some injections and also put her on a diet rich in Vitamin E, which has a powerful influence on the fecundity of women. These measures had no effect, and the unsatisfactory state of affairs continued.

Rather reluctantly, Henry, the husband, went to see his doctor – a practitioner whom he had been consulting for a good many years, and who naturally knew a good deal about his condition. He was not impressed by the suggestion that Henry might be infertile but under pressure he carried out certain microscopical and other tests, which established that there was no particular reason why, with a normal mate, Henry should not be the father of children.

'It's something we just have to face,' remarked this doctor. 'Unfortunately, modern civilization tends to make people infertile, and we really know very little about why some apparently normal people are fertile and others aren't. Quite a lot of people go through the same experience, but they don't give up hope, and in the end the trouble seems to clear itself up spontaneously.'

This was quite unexceptional and no dispute over the advice could arise. Yet it failed to get to the root of the matter. Still, Henry and Maisie remained childless. They consulted other doctors but without success, until at last Maisie went to a friend of mine who acts as a consultant to the Maynard Clinic. He was, it seems, the first ever to raise the question of venereal disease at all seriously.

Maisie felt at first, that his close questions were a little impertinent. She had had no sexual relations outside her marriage, and the idea that Henry might be or might have been infected was ridiculous in her view, to say the least. She said so rather hotly. And then Dr Caspan pressed her further.

'Getting back to yourself,' he said, 'did you have any relations before marriage?'

She admitted that she had had, though very occasionally.

'You never had any reason to suspect venereal disease?' he asked.

'Of course not. They weren't that kind of men, anyway.'

'Probably not. But you'd be surprised what kind of man is found to be suffering from venereal disease,' he commented. 'Well, it's only a forlorn hope, as I see it, but it's the only thing left. Sterility is an abnormal condition in any healthy human being. I can see no reason why you or your husband should be sterile. So I'm going to suggest you go along and see Dr Miles at the Maynard Clinic. I'll send you there privately, of course, and as Jonathan Miles is a friend of mine you need not trouble about anything.'

Maisie spent some time thinking it over. She knew pretty well what the signs and symptoms of venereal disease were, and she racked her memory to recall if she had ever had anything that vaguely resembled any of them, but without success. She trusted Dr Caspan, but she felt that his advice was even less than he had described it; it was not so much a forlorn hope as a desperate gesture from a man in complete bewilderment. She knew, too, that Henry would be outraged if she mentioned the matter to him.

When she reported on the affair to her husband, therefore, she merely said that she had been advised to see a specialist at the Maynard Clinic and left it at that. She found some irony in the fact that Henry, in ignorance of the full position, pressed her to overcome her reluctance and come to see me.

So it was by a very roundabout route that Maisie came to my consulting rooms. From the very first, she made it quite clear that she thought it was a waste of her time and mine, and that the suggestion was ridiculous.

'The more I think of it,' she said, 'the more absurd and impossible it seems.'

'Yet it is a possibility,' I pointed out. 'Even remote possibilities sometimes turn into actualities, especially in this branch of medicine. Your sterility is a fact. For a fact there must be some explanation or several alternative explanations. Everything else has apparently been excluded, so there remains venereal disease as a possible explanation of the sterility. I recommend, then, that you let me carry out a full examination.'

Though I pressed her hard, she could remember nothing at all helpful. But absence of evidence does not deter a VD specialist; he is too used to it – and for different reasons. He knows that in some cases there is literally no evidence, nothing to be seen, nothing experienced by the patient – or, at worst, nothing that might not much more readily come from some other cause. He knows, too, that patients' memories are notoriously unreliable in these matters; they seem afflicted with what Freud calls purposive forgetting, since they feel that any admission is a reflection on them. I do not think that Maisie's ignorance was due to the latter cause, but one could never be sure; the human mind is capable of deceiving even its possessor.

The more likely cause of sterility, if it was venereal in origin, would be gonorrhoea, though syphilis could not be entirely excluded. The obvious thing, therefore, was to examine with gonorrhoeal possibilities foremost in mind, though with reserved judgement on syphilis.

This was a case that bristled with difficulties. To all intents and purposes I was being asked to give an opinion on a perfectly healthy human being who honestly had no cause to believe she had been exposed to venereal infection. Moreover, if a gonorrhoeal infection was present, it would be very difficult to detect. Except in grossly acute cases, there is always some difficulty in diagnosis where women are concerned and, when the disease is of some standing, as this, if present, was likely to be, those difficulties become increased immeasurably.

'This is the position,' I said when I had questioned her closely without obtaining any helpful or illuminating answer. 'You've come to me as a last resort. It's impossible for me to say whether or not your sterility is due to venereal disease without my making an elaborate and probably protracted examination. I can make certain tests, but, taking all the circumstances into consideration, it's highly probable that the first one will be quite uninformative – but that won't exclude the possibility. Are you willing to undergo all this?'

This was one of the very rare occasions when I did not press the case of complete examination. I must confess that, as to my colleague, the possibility seemed remote. Apart from the alleged sterility – which might be due to a dozen or more different causes – there was no venereal suspicion at all.

She did not speak for some time, but sat with an expression of deep thoughtfulness on her face. I could imagine how perplexing the problem must seem to her, and I could well believe that the apparent inability of the medical profession to help her except by wild goose chases such as this must have seemed almost incredible to her.

At last she looked up and spoke slowly.

'It's difficult to decide,' she said, 'but I think on the whole you had better do everything you think necessary. I really don't see how VD can possibly come into it, for apart from anything else I'm quite sure that if Henry had been playing the fool he'd have done something about it and I should have known about it. He cares for me too much to make me run any risks of that kind, and I know his outlook. So my decision is to carry on, simply because there seems nothing else left to do. There's one thing, though,' she added, meaningly.

'Yes?' I returned.

'Until you've something definite to report, I want to keep Henry out of this. He mustn't know. He just knows I've come to the Maynard Clinic but I haven't told him what for. I shall tell him I've got to have some tests and be vague about it. You see, if he knew he might start thinking things and – well, there might be problems.'

'Very well, that's your affair – for the time being,' I said. 'But I must insist on one thing, too. If by any outside chance these tests should indicate VD of some kind, then you must tell him so that he too can and must come for tests.'

'But, of course!' she exclaimed. 'That's only commonsense and playing the game, isn't it?'

I nodded. I wished everyone else took the same view of playing the game.

The examination I gave her was very thorough indeed, but it revealed nothing of any great significance. One or two things might have been considered suspicious, but it is no good allowing oneself to prejudge appearances, and, further, one always has to guard against seeing what one expects to see. As I expected, the diagnosis would have to rest entirely on laboratory tests, but these again would be difficult. It would be quite in accordance with the case such as this might be, for the secretions I collected to give no significant indication at all.

So, in point of fact, it turned out. The bacteriologist could give no more than a vague report. The trouble with old infections, as this would be if it existed, is that other micro-organisms closely resemble the gonococcus, and even if gonococci themselves are present, they are in very small quantities only and may escape detection. But my patient and

I were determined to find out the truth if it was possible to do so, and accordingly I adopted 'provocative' measures by painting the parts of the body from which tell-tale secretions come with a solution of glycerine and pilocarpine. Twenty-four hours later, Maisie came back and again I collected samples. At the same time, I also took specimens of the blood. I did this for two reasons: the first, as a precaution, to test for syphilis; the second, so that I could apply the 'gonococcal complement fixation test', as it is called. This is on similar lines to the Wassermann test for syphilis, but it is far less reliable. It is, however, of special value where long-standing infection is suspected.

Rather to my surprise, this second series of tests all gave a positive reaction. To make doubly sure, the bacteriological department grew cultures from the secretions I had taken, and these gave the final piece of positive proof. Maisie was suffering from asymptomatic gonorrhoea of long standing. It was a surprising discovery which I had not expected to make; and I felt that the news was going to shock her terribly.

She took it with comparative calmness, though it was easy to see she was keeping herself well under control.

'I can't say this hasn't floored me,' she remarked. 'Has it surprised you?'

'In a way – yes,' I replied. 'I didn't expect it, but then things do sometimes turn out like this, and it isn't a doctor's business to be surprised at anything, however absurd it may seem at first.'

'I suppose not. Well, we can't run away from it,' she went on. 'Where do we go from here?'

'You'll have to undergo treatment – that's quite inescapable now,' I said. 'And you will have to talk to your husband and persuade him to come along here for examination. He may be able to throw some light on the affair.'

She sighed. 'Yes, I'll have to face it,' she observed. 'But I don't think he'll be able to explain it any more than I can.'

'That may be so. But there must be an explanation somewhere,' I rejoined.

Apparently she told Henry at once, for that very evening he rang me up and asked for an appointment. He made no comment on the telephone, but his voice was far from cordial. The day, when he came to see me, he was looking very determined and had very much the air of a man who had made up his mind to thrash out an awkward problem.

'I can't understand this, doctor,' he said in a forceful voice. 'Is it possible there's some mistake? I mean, it couldn't be something else? I'm not questioning your ability, but it's possible for the best of us to make mistakes sometimes.'

'I hardly think that arises,' I replied. 'I can understand that you find it very difficult to believe. But I, personally have checked the tests made in the laboratory by a bacteriologist of the highest standing, and I can say that the results are conclusive. The gonococcus is indisputably present. Moreover, the blood test confirms it.'

'Well I can't argue about that,' he said, obviously implying that he would if he could. 'What next?'

'I should like to have your wife here for forty-eight hours for penicillin treatment, and after that I shall want her cooperation in making sure that we've cured her. That is the first and urgent thing. I suggest she comes in today. I can arrange that.'

'Very well, then. I'll tell her and get her to ring you up to make the arrangements.'

'The next is that you also must undergo an examination.'

'Yes, I suppose so,' he observed with a doubtful air.

'And also I shall want you to try and help me to get to the bottom of this business.'

'I don't think I can help you,' he replied.

'You won't object to answering some questions?'

'No.' He still seemed doubtful and a little puzzled – so much so that I let him remain in thought for a little while. This was a happy thing to do, as it turned out, for he suddenly looked at me rather hesitantly and then proceeded to supply another surprise in a case full of surprises.

'I'm not sure that I can't help you,' he said slowly, 'though it seems ridiculous to me. I suppose I ought to tell you.'

'If there's anything you think would help me you certainly should tell it to me – for your own sake and your wife's,' I replied. 'What is it? Have you any history of VD?'

He stared at the floor.

'I suppose you expect it,' he returned. 'Well, there is, as a matter of fact. But it was so long ago.'

'This is important,' I remarked, 'Tell me all about it.'

'It doesn't seem to be important,' he said, still reluctant. 'I don't see how it can be anything to do with this. It was when I was only a kid really. I was eighteen then, and I'm forty this year, so it's about twenty years ago. Surely there couldn't be any connection.'

'There certainly could,' I rejoined. 'What was it? Did you have treatment? And what happened?'

He told me. He had left school at the end of the spring term, and he was not going up to Oxford till the following autumn. That summer he had a gay time, as he put it. He had every opportunity of doing whatever took his fancy, for his family was quite well-to-do; he had a small car of his own; and his father was one of the school that believes a youth should sow his wild oats and get that operation over as soon as possible. With his not inconsiderable amount of money and his charm, he quickly became embroiled with a somewhat fast set; and before long he found that he was suffering from gonorrhoea.

'It was a bit of a blow to me,' he remarked. 'Somehow one does not expect that sort of thing to happen to oneself. Of course, I went off to a doctor and he decided to treat me himself. He knew the old man was pretty well off and had a name to keep up and all the rest of it and he said he didn't want to cause the family any pain or unnecessary embarrassment.'

Those were the days before penicillin and other antibiotic drugs were available, and treatment of gonorrhoea was, in a sense, more difficult than the handling of syphilis. Add to that that his doctor was not a specialist, and it will be seen that young Henry was not in a very good state. The treatment, consisting principally of dealing with local conditions of the disease, took some time, which irked Henry – not unnaturally – and he grew impatient. At length, however, the treatment came to an end, and, after tests, Henry was pronounced completely cured.

'You weren't kept under observation?' I asked sharply.

'No. The doctor said I was OK and in any case if anything further developed I was to go straight back to him. But nothing did.'

'I see,' I commented, unable to keep the disdainful note out of my voice. In these days of sulphonamides and penicillin, most specialists think it desirable that patients should be kept under observation for at least six months after apparent cure, but even then a year's continual test and examination is not conclusive.

'And that was the end of it,' he said. 'Nothing else showed itself. The only thing was that I was scared stiff of women from that time on, and if you can believe me I never had anything to do with another one until I met Maisie and fell for her. You don't think it can be that, do you?' It was more a desperate appeal than a plain question.

'I'm not going to attempt to answer that question yet,' I replied. 'First of all, there are some more things I want to ask you. Did you go back to your friends – the people who had, I suppose, led you into this trouble?'

'No,' he replied. 'As a matter of fact, everything went upside down about that time. The old man had a car crash and it looked as though he wouldn't be able to do much any more – he was badly crippled. I was intended to go into business and later take over from him after I'd been to Oxford, but this put the cap on that. I had to cut out all ideas of going up and went straight into the office to get the hang of the ropes while the old man was still there to guide me. It was a good thing I did, too, for, three years later – that would've been when I'd've been coming down in the ordinary way – he pegged out. After-effects of the accident.'

'So you led a hard-working sort of life?' I asked.

'More or less. There was a fair amount of entertaining of customers to be done, so it wasn't too bad.'

'You mean drinks and dinners?'

He nodded. 'Yes. I know I wasn't very old for the job, but it had to be done, and if there was one thing the gang had taught me it was how to hold my drinks, so that didn't worry me.'

'I see.'

I went on to question him about possible symptoms of

recurrence. He was vague at first, but under leading questions he recalled quite a number of significant pointers. He had been much troubled by pains in his joints and had to give up tennis because of 'rheumatism' in his shoulders. But his father had had rheumatism, so he took no particular notice of it. And there were one or two other items that interested me.

When I had finished, he looked straight at me.

'Will you answer my question now, doctor?' he asked. 'I mean, whether I'm the cause of Maisie's infection?'

'I'll answer that after your tests,' I replied; and he gave me rather a hostile look.

It was no surprise to me to find that his tests were positive. The first series were conclusive. I told him so bluntly when he came to see me two days later.

'I'm having cultures grown,' I said, 'but only as a check. The other tests are quite sufficient in themselves. So you see now the answer to your question. You infected your wife.'

'I don't understand it,' he murmured completely bewildered.

'Then let me explain,' I went on. 'Your gonorrhoea was never cured in the first place. At the time you had it, the need for specialized treatment was even greater than it is today, and to discharge you on the strength of a single test was giving far too big a hostage to fortune. The main symptoms had been cleared up and what had happened was that a small circle of infection had been left in your body. You did quite a lot to help it to stay there – not deliberately but simply because you never had any proper advice.'

'How's that?' he asked in astonishment.

'You took up a life or had to take it up in which entertainment was an essential part,' I explained. 'You admitted by inference that you drank quite a lot. Now there's nothing like alcohol for putting the brake on treatment for VD. Now we use penicillin and other powerful antibiotic drugs, which are very, very effective, but even so we tell patients they must avoid alcohol for a month at least after treatment. You didn't have that advantage, and you should have kept off it for quite a long time. It wasn't your fault – I don't blame you. I'm only pointing out the facts.'

'They're far from pleasant,' he observed bitterly.

'They rarely are pleasant in these cases,' I said. 'Nor had you been warned if what forms possible recurrence might take. That's so, isn't it?'

'I expected it would be the same over again,' he answered.

'Very infrequently,' I commented. 'If you'd been told you'd've been off to a doctor – and preferably a specialist that time – as soon as you had the first twinge of those pains in the joints. It's a very strong pointer to chronic gonorrhoea.'

'I seem to have made a mess of things. It wouldn't be so bad if only I were concerned, but Maisie ...' He broke off, overwhelmed by his thoughts.

'The bright spot is that you're both under proper treatment now,' I remarked. 'And this time you won't make any mistakes. I shall put you under penicillin treatment at once, and you'll not be discharged until I've completely satisfied myself that everything has been cleared up.'

After the penicillin treatment, they were both kept under unusually strict surveillance. My own view is that after penicillin, six months is the longest period of observation necessary and even that is probably excessive; but Henry and Maisie remained under my eye for nearly a year. Then at last I let them go, giving them a number of warnings – which, so far as Henry was concerned, were unnecessary, for his experience had frightened him considerably.

'I suppose, doctor,' said Maisie, towards the end of the treatment, 'this puts finish to all our ideas of having children?'

'I can't see why it should,' I replied with a smile. I had been waiting for that aspect to turn up. 'There's no reason at all why you shouldn't. Of course, I don't claim that I've cured the sterility. All I can say is that if that still exists, it isn't due to concealed chronic gonorrhoea.'

'But isn't there anything we ought to do?' she asked.

'If you like,' I said, 'to make assurance doubly sure, come to me if you become pregnant, and I'll give you another course of penicillin. It isn't really necessary, but it's quite a wise precaution.'

'I will, doctor, I will.'

After they had left me, I reflected on their case. It was a

curious one in several ways and it taught some important lessons. The first was the unwisdom of entrusting the treatment of venereal disease to anyone but a specialist. It is true that today with antibiotic drugs, especially penicillin, cure is simply and safely effected, but the point here is that only the specialist can be trusted to diagnose venereal disease (especially gonorrhoea) and to say with such certainty as is possible that it is cured. The second point was that every case of venereal disease should, when discharged, be made to understand the forms in which it might possibly recur, so that he can at once come for examination if suspicions arise. Henry would undoubtedly have done so had he been informed of the significance of pains in the joints, but he had absolutely no reason to connect them with his previous condition. These are two points that are worth stressing in and out of season.

There is a postscript I can add to this interesting case. A little while ago I heard from Maisie. She telephoned the Clinic and asked me for an appointment. She was going to have a baby, she told me, and she wanted to act on my suggestion and have a further course of treatment. She is wise. I do not suppose for a moment that there is any chance of her infecting the child, but she will gain in peace of mind from the treatment. That will offset to some extent the worry and anxiety she had already suffered – those twin mental demons that are among the most tormenting offspring of the venereal diseases.

Case 10

ALFRED

The specialist in venereal diseases shares with specialists in other abnormal conditions a tendency to reflect how much easier his work would be, both in regard to the treatment of individual cases and in the larger sphere of general control, if only people would come to him for advice the moment any suspicious sign is noticed. This is no doubt true. If these ideal conditions were obtained in my own field there would be few if any cases of late syphilis, chronic gonorrhoea, or congenital syphilis, and we should be a long way further along the road that leads to complete public control of infection.

Yet in making that observation the specialist is taking a distorted view of the problem and failing to realize the peculiar difficulties of the layman. The small significant signs that mean so much to him do so precisely because he is a specialist; to the non-specialist – even sometimes to the general practitioner – they do not tell nearly so informative a story; and to the complete layman they simply mean nothing at all. If, on the other hand, tabulated lists of signs and symptoms were broadcast in detail, and the public exhorted to act as soon as any of them appeared, clinics would become choked with self-diagnosed patients who had not the remotest reason for being there, which, besides creating an immense amount of unnecessary work for the medical staff, would also create widespread mental torment and anxiety needlessly among perfectly innocent and infection free members of the community.

A sense of balance and proportion has to be observed in this, as in most things. Certainly, if a man or woman observes a gross syphilitic chancre after exposure to the clear risk of infection, and then does not come for treatment, that individual has earned nothing less than the greatest possible condemnation. But one cannot expect the ordinary person concerned with his own day-to-day affairs to suspect venereal disease when there has been no clear risk of contracting it on the appearance of, shall we say, a slight discharge that might easily be due to some quite innocuous cause. Nor can we be altogether harsh on him if he fails to see the association between one form of malaise and another and to realize that, together, they would immediately create the strongest suspicions in the mind of a man who, day after day for many years, has been examining cases of suspected venereal disease. Indeed, the specialist stands so near to his work that – let it be admitted – he is sometimes so unable to see it whole and in perspective that he will see a suspicious symptom where none actually exists! We are indeed fortunate today in possessing laboratory techniques of diagnosis that abolish the need for a decision to rest entirely on the opinion of the physician. So far as the venereal diseases are concerned, in fact, it is no longer possible for the doctors to disagree; they merely have to accept the cold, impersonal findings of the microscope and the serological reaction.

Some of these cases already described illustrate these points to a greater or lesser degree, but the one which follows will perhaps bring them out more clearly. It would be easy to say that Alfred should have added two and two together and made four of it – that he should have connected together his various ills and disabilities and immediately presented himself at the nearest VD clinic. He was not a venereal diseases specialist; and to extend the metaphor already used, so far as VD was concerned, he was in the state of a child who had never learnt that the symbol '2' stands for two, far less the fact that a pair of them are represented by the symbol '4'.

Alfred was a man of forty-five, and no different in his general background and circumstances from many thousands of others of his kind. Since the age of fifteen, when he had begun earning his living as an office boy, he had been employed by the same firm, with which he was now a stockkeeper. His education was neither better nor worse than that of most men in his position. On leaving his local school, he had taken a short course at a commercial college, where he had learnt shorthand, book-keeping, and allied subjects. He liked his evening glass of beer and a political discussion with his cronies in the local public house; his reading extended little further than the daily, evening and Sunday newspapers, with perhaps an occasional book of the lighter kind from the public library.

In his profession he had advanced steadily but unspectacularly, for he believed in stability rather than what is usually called success. It was better to be sure of a modest pension, earned by faithful service, than to rocket up to dizzy heights and come down like the stick. At the age of thirty-one he had decided that he wanted a home of his own instead of living in furnished rooms, and he had married a nice quiet woman, two years younger than himself, who for some years had worked in the dispatch department of his firm. They had had no children and, rather suddenly, his wife had died three weeks before her fortieth birthday. For three years he had been a widower – a widower who realized that he had lost a good wife, and whose experience of marriage had been so full of contentment that he was perfectly ready, a little later on, to consider entering again into the marital state. One says contentment rather than happiness because Alfred, typically, was one of those men to whom heavily supercharged words hardly seemed to apply; one could, for example, think of him as having borne his wife a very strong and loyal affection but never as having experienced the ecstasy and pains of passionate love.

This, then was Alfred – sober, solid, hard-working, reliable, respectable and respected as a good, if not very brilliant, fellow. He was as unlikely a candidate for the VD clinic as it would be possible to find. And it was precisely because he took little interest in what he thought of as the wicked ways of the world and so never regarded their dangers as applying to him (if, indeed, he realized that there were such dangers) that when, at last he came into my hands he was in a very bad state indeed. The warnings that he might have had would perhaps have been sufficient for a more knowledgeable man, but he could hardly be blamed for not heeding the cryptic messages of the oracle when he did not even realize that the oracle was speaking.

Alfred's troubles – or at any rate this phase of them – began when he found that his sight was becoming rather weak. Up till then he had enjoyed perfectly good vision and had never troubled to have his eyes tested. There was nothing remarkable about that, he thought. He remembered reading somewhere that the majority of people needed to use glasses for reading when they got older than forty; it was something to do with the hardening of the muscles with age that did something to the focus. He did not understand the technical details, but both what he had read and his own experience suggested that there was nothing abnormal in signs of weakening sight. It was just one of the things he must expect at his age. And, so far as general principles go, he was on perfectly safe ground.

A colleague at the office recommended an optician to him, and the following Saturday afternoon he went along. The test, which was entirely novel to him, fascinated him, though he had not the vaguest idea of what it was all about. His notion of eye-testing was that one simply tried on various pairs of spectacles until one found those which enabled one to read better, but it was all very impressive, and he felt that he ought to have his vision completely restored after all these proceedings.

The optician was a young man. He was good at his job but he was also honest enough to realize his limitations and to understand that he was only a refractionist and not an ophthalmic specialist. He looked up from his note-pad and smiled in a professional way that would have done credit to Harley Street.

'I think, sir, you ought to go along to the eye hospital or see a specialist,' he said.

Alfred was shaken abruptly out of his happy dreams of recovered perfect sight.

'Why?' he asked in his rather flat, self-effacing voice. 'There's nothing seriously wrong, is there? I mean, there's no risk of my going blind?'

From his childhood, one of his chief terrors had been blindness.

The optician shook his head. 'Nothing serious that I can see. As regards your vision, it's very good indeed for your age. There's a certain amount of what we call old sight, but that's only to be expected at your age, sir, and that's quite easy to put right with proper glasses.' He picked up his ophthalmoscope. 'You see this instrument?' he asked, with the air of a lecturer. 'This enables us to see inside the eye itself and find out whether it's healthy or not. I must confess there's an appearance inside your eye that puzzles me. That's why I think you would be wise to see a specialist or go to the hospital. I can give you a letter in either case.'

'I don't expect it's anything,' said Alfred, to whom any sort of ill-health was unthinkable. 'Perhaps I'm a little run down. That often affects the eyes, doesn't it? Besides, if I need glasses I must have been straining my eyes.'

'Yes, of course, sir,' said the optician, 'but I don't think it's anything of that sort. I do think very strongly you should go to an eye specialist. It's better not to take risks.'

'I'll think about it,' said Alfred, who could be quite obstinate when he chose. 'You make the glasses for me, and I'll see how I get on with them. Then if I have any trouble later on, I'll come and see you again.'

'Very well, sir,' said the optician, feeling that he had done his best. 'But I do want to impress on you that I advise you to go to a specialist.' He wanted to make quite sure that Alfred did not misunderstand him.

'Oh, I'm sure you're doing your best,' said Alfred, a little patronizingly.

He chose a pair of spectacle frames, had his face measured for them, and went on his way, with the information that he would receive a postcard when the glasses were ready and he was to call for them and a further exhortation to see the oculist ringing in his ears.

Alfred did not see an oculist. He did not dismiss the matter out of hand, for that was not his way, but he abided by his former decision to wait, all the same. He had his new glasses and he could certainly see better. He was experiencing no particular discomfort or pain in his eyes, and he felt perfectly fit. And there was the additional point that his insurance society was not one of those which paid optical benefit; so if he got into the hands of an eye hospital or an oculist he did not know whether the National Health Service will pay for all that and he was not inclined to spend more than was absolutely necessary.

These factors were to him unanswerable. The young optician was, he felt, probably being over-cautious; an older and more experienced man would have seen that there was nothing at all wrong. Young men always were inclined to get jumpy and try to show off how clever they were. Yet he would have been saved a lot of subsequent trouble if he had followed the eminently sound and honest advice of the optician.

A little while later, he found himself developing signs of what he thought was rheumatism. The pains were vague and affected his legs and back chiefly, and he told himself that middle age was making its mark at last. Well, that was no more than he must expect. At last the pains became quite violent, and reluctantly he decided to see his firm's doctor.

Alfred, of course, went as a panel patient, and his doctor was the most popular in the district. The waiting room was crammed with patients when he arrived, and he had to stand up. It was over an hour before his turn came, and he found the doctor worried, tired, and depressed with overwork. It was already past his time to start his round and there were still another dozen patients waiting. But he listened attentively to Alfred's recital. It was probably sciatica, he thought, and he would have liked to have carried out a full examination, but time was too short. The best thing was to send the man to the hospital.

'I'm going to send you to the hospital,' he said, pulling a piece of letter paper towards him. 'I think it's probably sciatica, but I'd like to have you properly overhauled.'

'Is it really necessary?' asked Alfred.

'It's the best possible course,' replied the doctor.

He gave Alfred the letter. Alfred went away. There seemed a conspiracy to get him into hospital, and he was more than reluctant to go. The office was very busy, for one thing, and he could not afford the time. If the doctor thought it was sciatica – though it should be noted, in fairness to the doctor, that he put forward that suggestion as little more than a guess – then that was good enough for Alfred. There was no need to go to hospital, where he would probably be prodded and pushed about by students, and they would want to try one of these high-falutin' experimental treatments on him. He threw the letter into the waste-paper basket and decided to let things go for the time being. The only thing he did were to purchase some liniments and medicated wadding from the chemist. The pains persisted, but he believed that they were a trifle easier.

Alfred had had two warnings, which, for a variety of reasons he did ignore. The fates had not been kind to him in letting him go to his doctor on a day when that unhappy man, like most general practitioners, was pressed almost beyond the limit of human endurance; for it is fairly certain that if he himself had thoroughly examined Alfred, checked on his pains, and heard the story of the eyes (which he would no doubt have examined for himself), he would have seen a warning light. These premonitions were unnoticed. It was the third that brought the matter to a head – and Alfred eventually to the Department for the Treatment of Venereal Diseases of the Maynard Clinic.

He continued with his self-prescribed treatment of his pains, without much success – which was hardly surprising. His sight grew worse, despite the glasses, and he began to notice a difficulty in raising the lid of his right eye, so that his colleagues at the office started to make weak jokes about it.

Odd things began happening to him. On his way back from the station after work one evening, he decided to take a short cut which led him through an unlighted alley between two blocks of flats. The way was quite familiar to him, for it was his normal route during the summer, but in the winter, with the dark evenings, he usually avoided it. There had been a robbery or two along that alley, and Alfred was, if not a timid man, a cautious one.

About half way along he suddenly felt a complete loss of direction. This was the darkest spot, which the light from the lamps at either end did not reach. It seemed to Alfred that his legs were failing him and that he could not stand up. Panic came over him, but he checked the impulse to cry out for help; he hated making a fool of himself in public. So he clung to the wall and felt his way gingerly along. Never had he welcomed anything so much as the lamplight gleaming at the far end. It seemed to restore him completely, for he walked along rapidly until he reached his house. His landlady brought his dinner in and commented that he was a little late. He did not explain to her what had happened; but merely said that he had made a call on the way from the station.

The adventure alarmed him a little, and he started to think that something must be wrong with him, but decided, in his usual way, to give it a little more time, to see how matters developed. His opinion was that he was run down, and rest over the week-end would cure him. When, a week later, he stumbled upstairs rather badly, and thereafter found himself gripping the baluster firmly on every staircase he negotiated it did not look as though his theory had much to recommend it.

Events were moving fast now in the mysterious processes that were affecting Alfred, but he was quite unable to interpret the warning signs that kept reaching him; and when the crisis came, it was external action, not his own, which forced him where he should have been long ago – in hospital.

Though, by now, he was feeling thoroughly unwell, Alfred continued to go to work. He was tormented by headaches and by sharp pains in his limbs, particularly the legs, that struck with the intensity of lightning. The dark was a torture to him, for he found increasing difficulties in keeping his balance. Several times, his manager tried to induce him to see a doctor, but he refused. Like many another man in his position, he was terrified of what might happen to him if he were laid up in hospital for any length of time. He was getting on in years and he could not run risks with his job, for he knew how difficult it would be for a man of his age to secure another. In this attitude he reflected one of the tragedies of our civilization, which forces men and women to regard preserving their employment as more important than the health of their own bodies.

Then one day, as he sat at his desk, he was suddenly

doubled up with abdominal pains. He felt he wanted to curl up into a ball like a hedgehog and he found himself gasping for breath. The manager and another man carried him into the former's office, and a doctor was sent for. This time the decision on whether or not medical advice was to be sought did not lie with Alfred – and in this lay his ultimate salvation.

The pains were so intense that Alfred could give little account of himself to the doctor, who had, therefore, to make a diagnosis from the external signs – always a difficult business, since it is the subjective symptoms which enable one to differentiate between various closely similar states. The doctor not unnaturally believed that it was appendicitis. An ambulance was sent for, and Alfred, too weak and suffering to protest even if he had wished to, was brought to the Maynard Clinic. There he was immediately X-rayed and a team of expert diagnosticians went to work on him.

This was the stage at which I was sent for by my colleagues. Dr Thornton gave me a brief outline of what he knew.

'The patient was sent in as a probable appendix,' he said, 'and these superficial appearances suggest it. But the X-ray doesn't entirely bear it out, and there's no temperature. He couldn't talk much when he came in, but he's better now and has given me a few facts. I think this is your line of country, Miles. Looks to me like a clear-cut tabes dorsalis.'

Alfred was removed to my department, as Thornton had suggested, where I had him put in a small ward. All the appearances, of course, suggested tabes dorsalis – perhaps better known as locomotor ataxia – which is one of the more distressing results of neuro-syphilis. The state of his eyes was characteristic; they had what are called Argyll-Robertson pupils, which are completely insensitive to light changes and remain fixed, instead of varying in size as the light glows brighter or dimmer, yet they are capable of altering their focus to see objects at various distances. Moreover, they were abnormally small, though the right was a little larger than the left, and the circumference of the pupils, instead of being circular, had a slightly irregular edge. The eye-lids drooped noticeably – an effect due partly to mild paralysis of the muscles and partly to an attempt to compensate for the loss of light reaction in the pupils.

When he had recovered a little more under treatment designed simply to relieve his violent internal pains and consisting of simple analgesic drugs, I had him out of bed and asked him to walk. His gait, however, was not so typical of his suspected condition as the other symptoms might have suggested. The tendency to walk with feet wide apart and to lift the feet high in the air, jerking them forward, and ending the action with a pronounced stamp, was only slight. All the same, it was sufficient to be highly significant to me.

Already I was practically certain in mind, and so it was that the confirmation provided by tests of the blood and cerebro-spinal fluid was not at all surprising. Alfred must have had tertiary syphilis for some time, though it would be impossible to attempt to find out the history of the case until he was generally in better condition.

Tabes dorsalis is, essentially, the same as GPI, only the parts of the body affected differing between one state and the other; that is to say, it arises from infection of the central nervous system by the spirochaetes. The treatment therefore follows much the same course with, today, penicillin and some other antibiotic drugs as the chief weapon in the armoury of attack. Local treatment has, too, to be applied in many cases to restore the action of the muscles that have become paralysed to a greater or a less extent. In Alfred's case there was not much involvement of this kind, but he was given routine massage treatment and exercises to enable him to walk more easily again.

At last I was able to reach what is always for me the most interesting aspect of all venereal cases – the story that lies behind the infection. The variety of ways in which individuals acquire the diseases presents the most difficult of all problems to solve if we are to bring this scourge under full control. Today – it cannot be too often stressed – the medical aspect has been reduced almost to a routine with results that are practically always successful. It is only by obtaining every possible fact about the background of each and every case that we can secure sufficient data on which to base constructive planning for the final assault.

Alfred was not an easy patient to talk to. He was dominated by a sense of guilt and shame, and he did all he could by evasions and other means to sidetrack the issue. At one time, indeed, I was afraid that he was developing hysterical symptoms – sudden recurrence of attacks of pain and the like whenever the subject of his case history was mentioned. There was no physical cause for these attacks; they were hysterical attempts to avoid discussing something that was most unpleasant to him and the very mention of which gave him a feeling of intense guilt. This was a situation that had to be firmly handled. It was lucky that he was under close observation, for the tendency could be nipped in the bud. I was intentionally retaining him in the Clinic, for I had every reason to suspect that, if he was allowed to go free, his guilty feeling might induce him never to return. Even more than most other diseases, VD is hedged about by all manner of psychological complications.

But one day he brought the subject into the open on his own initiative – or, rather, he tried to kill it once and for all.

'When I'm discharged from here, I suppose I shall be completely cured?' he asked.

I nodded reassuringly. 'Yes,' I replied, 'you can take that for granted, though, as I've already told you, I shall want you to come back to me at intervals so that we can make sure that nothing has been overlooked. You came here just in time. If it had been left a little longer, your sight might have been permanently affected, and you might have had trouble with your legs for the rest of your life.'

'There's no doubt that it was – it was what you said it was?' he inquired. This was typical of his psychological state; he could not bring himself even to mention the words that increased his sense of guilt.

'None at all,' I replied. 'But that's nothing to worry about. The great thing is that we've been able to cure you before irreparable harm was done.'

For a minute or two he was silent.

'Then doesn't that finish it, doctor?' he asked at last with an obvious effort. 'It doesn't matter how I got it or anything of that sort, does it?'

I'm afraid I can't agree with that,' I returned. 'So far as you are concerned, the case is over. But in this world we've other people to consider. You don't want anybody else to go through what you've experienced, I'm sure. You wouldn't wish it to your worst enemy. So you see we ought to try to find out how you got it so that, perhaps, we can check another source of infection. Where you got it, someone else possibly could as well – and that means more trouble and more suffering. You can see that, can't you?'

'Yes,' he said slowly, 'I suppose that's true. But if I did tell you, you wouldn't go and force someone else to come here?'

'Unfortunately, no one has the power, as a general rule, to force anyone to take treatment for venereal disease,' I answered. 'If you worked here for a little while, you'd probably come to think that that was a very unsatisfactory state of affairs. You might be able to induce someone else to come for examination, but even then we could not insist on treatment, however bad the case might turn out to be. Putting that aside, though, there's another aspect. The more we know of how these diseases are spread, the better we shall be able to fight them, and make it safer for other people. That means studying individual cases. You can see that, can't you?'

He said no more on that occasion, but I lost no opportunity of making indirect appeals to him, and in the end he began to tell his story hesitatingly. Often he would break off and abruptly change the subject. It was clear that he had immense moral and psychological barriers to overcome, and in some ways our conversations tended to resemble psycho-analysis in which resistances had to be dispersed.

A great deal of his story I have already told in the earlier parts of the chapter, which is based on these talks, but I have held back to this stage his own narrative of how he became infected. Like so many of the narratives I had heard, it was pitiful enough.

'After my wife died,' he said in his flat, precise, yet self-effacing voice, 'I was very lonely, doctor. She was a very good wife to me, and I feel very much ashamed that I have disgraced her memory like this.

'You need not worry about that,' I interposed.

'That is how it seems to me and will always seem to me, doctor,' he observed primly. 'It was torture to know what to do. I hated going back to the empty house every evening after work. I had a daily help to do the work for me, you see and she stayed to give me my evening meal. But after that I was alone. I thought the best thing I could do was to sell up the place and go into apartments, like I had lived before, but against that I did not like the idea of getting rid of her things and letting them fall into the hands of strangers. It was a very distressing problem, doctor – very distressing.'

Silently, I noted that this was an attempt to avoid coming to the point, yet, at the same time, it was interesting as casting a side light on a rather pathetically indecisive personality.

'In the end,' he continued, 'I compromised. I decided to go into rooms, but not to sell the furniture for the time being. I took a few things for my own use, and put the rest into store. It was expensive, but I felt that it was for the best. I thought that later on I might feel like setting up home again, and then the furniture and other things would be very useful. I found quite comfortable quarters, and for a little while I was quite contented. But I was still very lonely, doctor. It was a very terrible thing to be lonely.'

'Loneliness,' I rejoined rather tritely, 'is the great curse of modern big towns.' I might have added that it was probably the ultimate driving force that sent men and women out on adventures that, in the end, brought them to VD clinics up and down the country; but I thought it wise not to say so to him.

'About a year after Clara died,' he resumed, after a brief pause, 'it – this – happened.' It was the usual characteristic hesitation. 'At least, I suppose it was then, now I know what you've told me. You see, I still went occasionally to have a drink in the evenings. It was company of a kind, though I rarely spoke to anyone. I liked to have people about me and to see people enjoying themselves. I wish now I had found company elsewhere.'

'You can never tell where danger lies,' I commented.

'That is very true, doctor – very true, indeed. I suppose you see a lot of that. It must be heart-breaking for you.'

'What happened?' I asked.

Again he paused. When he spoke it was with a distinct effort.

'One night in a public house,' he went on, 'I was sitting in a corner, listening to the talk, and a woman came and sat next to me. I can't say I noticed her very much. Then she began talking to me – nothing much, so far as I can remember. Probably about the weather and things like that. She was a pleasant-looking woman, not too young, quietly dressed – I imagined her probably a widow who let rooms or something like that. I was very lonely.'

He kept insisting on this point as though it was the one, over-riding excuse for everything that happened.

'She was very sympathetic and understanding,' he continued, regathering his courage and gulping a little, 'and in the end I bought her a drink. We had got on very well together, and when she left I promised to look out for her again. Well, in the end, I told her about my affairs – it was nice to have someone to talk to – and she seemed to understand my position exactly. She invited me round the following Saturday afternoon to have a cup of tea with her. I accepted. I could see no harm in it, and I thought it would make a very pleasant change.'

Little beads of perspiration were standing out on his forehead. Recalling all these events was an exquisite mental torture to him.

'On the Saturday I went – and I really can't say what came over me,' he resumed, speaking more quickly now, as though anxious to see the matter finished as soon as possible. 'She entertained me lavishly, doctor, as though I were an honoured guest. I stayed to supper and then – then' – he passed his hand across his damp brow – 'then she suggested to me I might as well stay the night. No one need know, she said – she was alone in the house – and in any case it was time I had a few home comforts again.'

It was difficult to suppress the smile that this statement roused in me, but he was in sore distress and it would have been cruel, perhaps dangerous, to let him think he was being ridiculed.

'I'm ashamed to say that I fell,' he continued. 'I saw her regularly after that. She told me that she led a very hard life and was in financial difficulties, and of course, I was only too glad to help her. I didn't think anything of it that her difficulties never seemed to clear up and I barely noticed that I was giving her money every time I saw her. I was beginning to dip into my little savings, but then I felt it was all in a good cause. We got on so well together I begun to consider that we might marry. In fact, I even raised the question once in a vague sort of way.'

He gripped his hands together tightly.

'She began crying when I mentioned it,' he said. 'She said her husband had left her a long time ago and there had never been a divorce, and he couldn't be found. I told her I was sorry and let the matter drop. I suppose I should have gone on seeing her, if something else hadn't happened. It was a terrible shock to me.'

'Tell me about it,' I urged softly.

'Yes, doctor, but it is a terrible thing to have to talk about,' he murmured. 'You see, if I didn't go straight to her house, I always met her in the public house where I had first seen her. I rarely went anywhere else. You know how it is about your own local. One night, though, I was late home from the office, and I decided I'd like a drink before I went back, so I dropped in to a public house near the station – one I didn't often go to. Almost the first thing I saw was Maggie – that was her name. I was going to speak to her when I saw she had a man with her. They seemed on very intimate terms. I don't know why, but I tried to keep out of sight among the crowd, and I don't think she saw me. And then when she left with the man, I slipped out and followed them. Of course, they went to her house. I waited for a little while and then I saw the light go out in the dining-room and the light switched on in the bedroom on the floor above. I could see their shadows on the blind.' He dropped his head in his hands. 'It was horrible!' he said in a barely audible voice.

'It must have been a great shock to you,' I said colourlessly.

'I felt as though I was going mad,' he returned. 'I didn't know what to do. But worse was to come. I was supposed to meet her the next evening but I felt I couldn't. But all the same I went down to the public house. I went into the public bar instead of the saloon, where we always met, and I managed to get glimpses into the saloon. She was there, sitting in the usual place. After a little while, she went out, looking rather angry. I gave her a minute or two, and then I went out too. She was walking down the road, looking about her, and I followed her. She went down to a part that had rather a bad reputation behind the station. I saw her go into a public house and I waited. She came out quite soon, and then she began walking up and down smiling at men. I felt sick, doctor, and when at last she spoke to a man and they went off together after a little talk, I thought I was going to faint. She was nothing more than a common prostitute, I suppose, and she'd got round me like she had because she'd realized I wouldn't have even spoken to her if I'd known the truth. Oh, it was terrible!'

I said something consoling and reassuring.

'And you think she infected you?' I asked at last.

'It couldn't be anything else,' he replied in a pleading tone. 'I've never had anything else to do with women since then. It was too much of a shock anyway. If that man she picked up down there was the sort she went with, she must have been rotten.'

'And you never noticed anything on yourself – or on her?' I pressed.

He was silent again. His readiness to talk about the general situation did not extend to his own personal details. But at length the truth came out. Yes, about that time he had noticed 'a small sore', it had not seemed to him important.

'It soon cleared up when I put some ointment on it,' he said.

The old story – the 'self treatment' that leads to so many disasters and sometimes makes the difficulties of accurate diagnosis much worse.

He had noticed nothing else. The secondary stage, so far as I could find out, had not been at all marked – which is not unusual; and it was clear from the condition in which he had been brought to hospital that the micro-organisms had made rapid progress in their attack on his system. The events he described to me had occurred about two years earlier. Now it is possible for symptoms of neuro-syphilis to appear as early as and concurrently with the secondary stage, when the infection begins to spread throughout the body, but in the main they show themselves not less than a year, and more frequently much later – sometimes as much as fifteen years or more, taken from the time of infection. Premonitory symptoms had appeared, though not in a form he would recognize and indeed no one would at once recognize except as suspicious indications in cases of admitted infection – neurosthenic headaches and vague pains.

I asked him if he would look up the woman concerned and try to induce her to come for an examination. The inference was that, unless she had had treatment meanwhile, she was still spreading the disease. As I expected, he refused. This was one of the few occasions on which he showed real firmness of decision.

'Nothing at all would ever persuade me to see her again,' he said. 'I feel sick at the mere thought of her. I don't doubt the other men who go with her know her for what she is, and they must look after themselves.'

Superficially he was a mild, inoffensive man, but from the way in which he said that and from other unintentional hints he gave me, I think he derived some psychological satisfaction from the thought that others were falling as he fell and sharing his punishment. It helped him to believe that his guilt, which was so strongly marked, was not unique.

That was all I was able to extract from him. I have set the story out here as a connected narrative, but in actual fact it was not told me in that way. He gave me the story in many instalments, now adding one detail now another, until, in the end, I had obtained a pretty clear picture; and I think, too, that he gained some sort of relief by the mere act of confiding in someone.

There is little more to add to the history of his case. I retained him under observation in the Clinic as long as I decently could for I wished to make sure that even if he did not return for routine examination he was reasonably safe; and also I hoped to relieve him of some of his sense of guilt and shame so that his resistance to returning could be reduced. In this I was partially successful. He did come regularly for about nine months, but after that he disappeared. I tried to get in touch with him at the address he had left and also at his place of work; but in each case I drew a blank. He had gone away, no one knew where. At his lodgings, a couple of letters had been waiting for him for several weeks.

Alfred was quite cured – I am certain of that as anyone could be in such a case; and I do not think that his experience left any permanent physical mark on him. But I am equally sure that the psychological effects would be more lasting and perhaps be with him for the rest of his life. This is an important but not often discussed, aspect of venereal diseases, but it cannot be entered into here. I can only say, and I shall develop the theme a little later on when I come to speak generally of the problems of control, that this particular effect is bound up with the false general attitude to venereal disease. Those who approach the subject rationally are not likely to suffer any lasting psychological harm. Nevertheless, the VD specialist has always to bear in mind the development of neurotic and even psychotic complications and occasionally he has to call in the help of the psychiatrist to ensure that a perfectly healthy individual is sent back into the society of his fellows.

One other sidelight of the difficulties of handling venereal disease suspects was brought out by this case, but only in an incidental way and as the result of a rather unusual proceeding on my part.

While Alfred was with us I happened to notice the name of the optician on his spectacle case, and I idly asked him if that was the man who had told him he should see a doctor on the occasion of the eyesight test. He had replied that it was.

A little later I made up my mind to see the optician, for I was interested to find out if he had any suspicions, and, if he had, why he was not more definite.

I found the shop, which was one of the branches of a large firm. Very courteously, they turned up their records and found that the optician who had tested Alfred's eyes had been moved to another shop, where he was now manager. I thanked them and sought out the new address.

Mr Price, the optician, I found to be an extremely capable and serious-minded man, who took his job with real professional pride. He remembered Alfred's case quite well when he had been given a few details to refresh his memory.

'Tell me,' I said, 'when you suggested he should see a doctor, had you anything definite in mind?'

He nodded slowly, but said nothing.

'You need not be afraid to talk,' I observed. I told him my status and that Alfred was one of my patients.

'Oh!' he exclaimed. 'So it was that!'

'You did suspect it, then?'

Again he nodded. 'Yes,' he replied. 'The optic disc was pale and had a sort of chalky appearance. It puzzled me a little at first, and as soon as I could after he'd been to see me, I looked it up. The only description I could find that tallied was syphilis.'

'You said nothing to him?' I demanded.

He shook his head. 'I was as insistent as I could that he should see a specialist or go to the hospital. I couldn't go further than that. If I'd told him he might have got very nasty, you know. People don't like being told things like that – especially by men who aren't doctors – and,' he added with a slight smile, 'I don't suppose some of them like it even when you tell them.'

'They don't,' I said feelingly. 'Definitely not.'

'I suppose,' he went on reflectively, 'I ought to have been more definite with him and dropped a strong hint. But my position was very difficult. I was on my first job, then, and I wasn't too sure of the ropes, and I wasn't looking for trouble with customers or with my employers either. He'd come to me to have his eyes tested, and I prescribed glasses to correct his refractive errors. Strictly speaking, my job ends there. People come to see me to consult me about their sight – their health is their doctor's business.'

'Yes, I suppose that is the strict position. I know there's no love lost between my profession and yours, but for myself I don't see why there need be any fight, for after all, you people do a lot of good work that relieves the oculists of a great deal of trouble – and you do it very well. But now, after this case, do you still think you would act in the same way? Wouldn't you feel, if you saw the same appearance again in the ophthalmoscope, that you ought to move heaven and earth to get the man to hospital, as much for the public interest as for his own sake?'

'I hope it never happens,' he replied, 'because it'd put me in a hell of a jam. If it was anything else but VD, of course I'd press like blazes. But VD is a sort of taboo, isn't it?'

I thanked him, after a little more chat, and went away. He was right in his own way. VD, even now, is taboo still with most people and I imagine that a non-medical man, like an optician, who suggested it to a customer or client (whichever they call them), might in certain circumstances lay himself open to an action for slander. That seems to me one more argument why all engaged in medical and paramedical work, like sight-testing, should be under the same umbrella. But that is ranging far outside my subject. Nevertheless, the affair brought out yet one more problem to be faced in dealing with the general question of venereal diseases and their ultimate control.

Case 11

SCANDAL IN SCHOOL

All manner of people come to the Clinic, and one grows out of being surprised at the utter impartiality with which the venereal diseases strike. The rich and the poor, the clean and the unclean, the moral and the immoral; terrified people with already the lunatic asylum opening its doors for them; phlegmatic people who say simply that they 'asked for it, and they've got it' – all these and many more make up the case-books of the years. Nevertheless, I could not refrain from lifting my eyebrows slightly when my secretary told me that he had booked an appointment for a Miss Barbara Holiwell.

'Know anything about her?' I asked. 'Coming on her own or sent here by a doctor?'

With a slight smile – my secretary is a somewhat cynical young man – he handed me a visiting card.

'She called and wanted to see you at once – and she seemed in a hell of a flap,' he remarked nonchalantly, 'Most annoyed when I said you weren't here and couldn't be seen until tomorrow.'

I glanced at the card. Then it was that I lifted my eyebrows. 'Miss Barbara Holiwell, M.A. (Lond.), Headmistress,' I read, and below, the name of a girl's school in the southern half of England.

'That's all I know,' went on my secretary, gratified at my expression of surprise. 'Why she wants to see you, I don't know. Whether she's the patient or not, or whether she wants you to lecture to the girls, I don't know either. But she says it's quite urgent and she obviously thinks it's scandalous you weren't here to see her at once. I imagine she'll be tough.'

The card raised my interest. I knew nothing of Miss

Holiwell or her school. All I knew was that I'd never before had the headmistress of a girls' school wishing to see me urgently. Luckily I was too busy to speculate, and, in fact, I forgot the appointment until my secretary reminded me of it next morning. It was the first on my list.

Miss Holiwell turned out to be a somewhat austere-looking, aggressive woman in, I should say, the mid-fifties. She was severely dressed in a dark-blue costume that hinted, from its cut and air of weariness, that it had been a friend of some years' standing. When I induced her into my patient's easy chair, she sat bolt upright on the extreme front edge of the chair, with her hands folded in her lap.

'Yes, Miss Holiwell,' I said, when she was settled, 'now how can I be of assistance to you?'

She looked at me with a suspicion of disfavour.

'I wish to make one thing clear, quite clear, doctor,' she said, in an edged, reedy voice. 'I'm not here to consult you about myself. Most definitely not.'

'No,' I said. 'I am sure of it.'

'I have come to you, doctor,' she went on, with the air of one giving a carefully prepared lecture, 'because I am given to understand that you are a leading authority on – er – er – certain diseases.'

'I make no claim to being what you so·kindly term a "leading authority",' I replied, noting her evasion; it was a useful index to her attitude. Things like that count for much in showing how the interview must be subsequently shaped and developed. 'All I can say is that I have had considerable experience as a specialist in venereal diseases.'

She winced a little at my forthrightness, which was intentional.

'Quite so, quite so, doctor,' she said. 'I am also given to understand that you can be of assistance to me in a problem – a terrible problem – that has arisen in my school. I must confess I am overwhelmed by it.'

'One moment, madam,' I interposed. 'May I try to get things clear?

She inclined her head.

'Now. Twice you have said, "you are given to understand"

things about me. May I ask who has given you this information? And also may I ask you to state, as briefly as you can, the problem you wish to discuss with me?' I ostentatiously looked at my wrist watch. 'I am extremely busy today – I hope you will forgive my mentioning it.'

'How terrible that sounds, doctor! I mean, of course, that a specialist in your line should find so much to occupy him.' She was a little nonplussed by my deliberate hint that I was not going to have my time wasted. Schoolmasters and schoolmistresses, used as they are to positions of demi-deity, do not like being spoken to in that way. 'My school doctor – Dr. Balmer – has informed me of your work. This is the source of my information. As to the problem, it is a very terrible one. Dr. Balmer was called in to examine three of my girls – admirable girls in every way, doctor – and he finds them, so he says, to be in a state that seems to merit your attention. Since then, there have been further outbreaks.' She paused. 'I hestitate to use the word "epidemic" in this connection, but I am not sure that it would be entirely inapt.'

'And this "state", as you call it? May we have plain speaking, Miss Holiwell? It's no good beating about the bush.'

She moistened her thin lips and a look of horror crept into her eyes.

'Dr Balmer calls it, I think – now let me see.' She made an effort at memory – or was it to overcome moral distaste? 'He called it, if I remember rightly, vulvo-vaginitis.'

'Ah! I exclaimed, beginning to see daylight. 'Will you give me details first?'

'Very well, doctor,' she replied. 'It appears that this repellent state can be due to various causes, but Dr Balmer says quite definitely that this particular outbreak is caused by the same germ as – well, I suppose I need not tell you.'

This archness made me feel irritated.

'Do you mean that some girls in your school have been infected with gonococcal vulvo-vaginitis?' I asked, brutally.

She winced. 'That is the position,' she said severely. 'It is a most terrible situation, doctor. If it is true, it will be a most difficult thing to explain to parents – who, of course, will have to be informed that their girls are ill. It will also create most unworthy reflections on the school, doctor, if the news gets about. Nothing could be more distressing. Above all else I have always laid first emphasis on a high moral tone in my school, and that this should happen is disastrous.'

I felt sorry for her, for she was indeed facing an awkward situation. But I did not like her manner in the slightest. What troubled her was the damage to her school's reputation (with subsequent loss of fees, it might be) more than the sufferings of her pupils.

'Can you tell me whether Dr – er Dr Balmer has made any tests before reaching this conclusion?' I asked.

'He did, doctor. I strongly resented his first suggestion that this disease might be caused by what I believe you term gonococcal infection. I cannot say that his other possible explanations – uncleanliness and so on – were much less distressing. However, he took what he called samples, sent them to a laboratory, and then told me his suspicions were confirmed beyond doubt.'

'I see. Then that's quite definite,' I remarked. 'And now what do you want me to do?'

'I wish you to take the situation in hand,' she replied firmly. 'Dr Balmer enjoys my complete confidence, but I should like to have your specialist ruling on the matter. If you also confirm it, I shall ask you to apply the best possible treatment. You need not be afraid to name your fee.'

I could not resist a somewhat bitter smile. 'Of course, if you wish it, I will take the case in hand,' I said. 'As to the fee, if any that doesn't concern me. The National Health Service will provide for everything necessary for the treatment and you will have to discuss the matter with the Almoner of the Clinic. But do you really think my intervention is necessary? From what you have said, your own doctor has had his diagnosis confirmed by laboratory tests on sera, and I can do no more. As for treatment, no doubt he also seems perfectly competent to give that.'

'I have my reputation and that of my school to protect,' she answered fiercely. 'I can never let it be said that, in a crisis of this kind, I failed to seek the most authoritative advice. The situation is terrible enough without giving people the opportunity of saying that I remained complacent in the face of it.'

'Very well,' I said. 'What Dr Balmer says? He knows you've come to me, I take it.'

She nodded primly. 'Yes, doctor. I gather that he would be delighted to work with you.'

'Very well,' I said again. 'Now you must help me a little.'

'I am anxious to do all I can, doctor, however painful it may be to me,' she returned.

'Thank you. I do think it need not be at all painful, for it will only involve perfect frankness, Miss Holiwell,' I said. 'Now you must forgive me if I admit that I know nothing of your school. What sort of a place is it – I mean how many pupils have you and what are their ages?'

'We are a small private boarding school of the very highest class,' she replied, speaking as though she was quoting from her prospectus. 'We limit our numbers strictly to sixty, so that every girl shall have personal attention and be allowed to develop her own personality without the cramping that large numbers bring. Their ages range from ten to sixteen years. At the moment we have very few senior girls – the majority of our pupils are between ten and fourteen.'

'I see. Thank you,' I rejoined. 'That is a very clear picture. And I take it all are boarders?'

'That is so,' replied Miss Holiwell. 'We take no day girls. Their presence would upset the very carefully thought out curriculum of the school.'

'And where do your girls come from?'

'From the very best families, doctor,' she answered. 'Most of them are the children of parents who are overseas – in the Foreign Office Service and so on – and I have complete charge of them. You can understand that this is specially trying to me; it is essential that the matter be cleared up.'

'I see that.' I looked at her sharply. 'This may be an awkward question for you, madam,' I went on, 'but it is essential I should know. You have had no other trouble with any of the senior girls? No suggestion, for example that one of them might have been having sexual intercourse?'

Her mouth shut sharply like a trap.

'A ridiculous suggestion, doctor, if I may say so!' she protested. 'All my girls are under constant surveillance – the senior ones under my own personal supervision. And I can assure you that by the time they reach the sixth form, they have had their moral concepts so developed that nothing of that kind could happen. I make a point of getting rid of girls at an early stage who do not show signs of responding completely to the moral guidance they receive.'

'I see,' I remarked.

'That,' she continued, 'is one of the factors which make the situation so utterly incomprehensible. I was always under the impression that infections of this kind came only from the sort of loose behaviour you mentioned just now. That would be bad enough if only one girl was infected. But now, there are at least half a dozen other cases.'

'You can set your mind at rest,' I replied, rising and walking to the mantelpiece, where I rested my arm. 'Both the venereal diseases can be spread by other means than sexual intercourse, but the chances of its so occurring are slightest of all in gonorrhoea. Yet it does happen with young girls, and this particular form of it, vulvo-vaginitis, is the way in which it affects them, due to certain differences in tissue structure as between adults and children. Contact with an infected person, or with infected towels or clothing, is the means by which the children get it as a rule.'

'It is terrible, doctor!' she exclaimed. 'I do not think I need know anything more.'

'If you will excuse me, madam,' I returned, 'I myself feel that it is vitally important for a lady in your position to be acquainted with the facts of this condition. Here is a case very much to the point. It may be that had you been informed you might have anticipated the danger and averted it.'

'Are you accusing me of negligence?' she snapped, bridling.

'Nothing was further from my thoughts,' I replied. 'I am only suggesting that knowledge of all the possible dangers that may arise in, say, a school – even the most unlikely and remote ones – seems to me a very desirable thing. However,' I went on quickly, 'you wish me to handle the case. I suppose that means I shall have to come down to see Dr Balmer, for a start.

Shall I telephone him and make arrangements?'

'It will be sufficient if you tell me when you can come,' she answered.

'I will come tomorrow – about three o'clock, if that is convenient,' I said, after glancing at my appointments pad.

'Will it be difficult, doctor?' she asked.

'If you mean will it be difficult to treat, the answer is no,' I returned. 'In these days of penicillin and other antibiotic drugs, it is quite a simple and speedy matter, though it will be necessary to keep the patients under strict surveillance – medically – I mean for about six months to guard against possible relapse. But it will be more difficult, I fancy, to solve the bigger problem: how the girls were infected. You see, unless we do that, there is always the risk of reinfection.'

'I could not face another outbreak,' she said decidedly. 'I will do anything I can to avoid that. This will need the greatest care in handling, doctor, I need not ask you to be discreet.'

'Discretion,' I replied – not very happily, in the circumstances – 'is one of the first and most important things one learns in a VD clinic.'

She shot me a look of disgust and prepared to depart.

'I will expect you tomorrow, doctor. How will you come?'

'By road,' I replied.

She shook my hand and I showed her to the door.

The interview left me with mixed feelings of amusement and anxiety. Miss Holiwell's attitude had been almost ludicrous at times, and I pitied the unfortunate girls whose upbringing was entrusted to this mass of inhibitions, false modesty, prudery, and straitlaced morals. Yet it was certainly a serious position she was facing, for scandal in a girls school can be far more serious than the same thing in a boys' school. There were all manner of ways in which vulvo-vaginitis could have been introduced into the school, but it was no good speculating on them. I anticipated that, if I was to elucidate the truth of the matter, I was going to have a pretty trying time, for if Miss Holiwell had projected her own attitudes onto her assistants and her pupils, the last thing I could expect was a willingness to face facts frankly.

On my arrival next day at the school, I found the situation rather more serious than Miss Holiwell had suggested. I do not think that the understatement of the circumstances was deliberate on Miss Holiwell's part, for I think she would have rather been inclined to overplay her hand in an effort to impress me with the gravity of affairs. She was, however, totally ignorant of the nature of progress of the disease and so did not realize that some of the cases, of which there were now eleven in all, had developed very severe symptoms.

The history of the outbreak was given to me briefly by Dr Balmer whose attitude towards me was somewhat negative. He did not resent my presence; on the contrary he seemed a little relieved at having the burden of an unsatisfactory business thrown on to someone else's shoulders. At the same time, I could not help noticing that he regarded my being called in as rather unnecessary.

'Pity the old dear insisted on wasting your time,' he remarked. 'But that's her way. I've known her for some time, and to my mind she's one of the strongest arguments for the abolition of private boarding schools in this country. She wouldn't give two hoots if the little brats died so long as they did so without danger to her reputation and her income. That's one of the things that's made her panic, I think – the question of income. The school is rather empty just now, and she's all out for more pupils, so this business has come at a very awkward time.'

'I see,' I remarked colourlessly, not altogether interested in this mode of approach. 'D'you mind giving me the facts as briefly as you can? I want to get back as soon as possible.'

'I don't blame you,' he commented, and proceeded to outline the development of the outbreak.

He had been called one evening to examine one of the girls who had been taken ill with acute abdominal pains. At first he had suspected appendicitis, which is not unusual in severe attacks of this kind in the disease, but further examination had revealed that this was not the truth. The typical inflammation of vulvo-vaginitis was only too evident, and Balmer, who, for all his assumption of cynicism and indifference, was really a good doctor, insisted on a general examination of all the pupils. The result were somewhat shocking. Counting the girl to whom he had been called, he found seven cases in all, showing signs of the disease in a more or less severe form, and since then there had been four more cases, one diagnosed as recently as the previous afternoon when Miss Holiwell was delivering herself of her troubles to me.

Balmer's conduct had been unexceptional. He had taken sera from all the infected girls and made arrangements for the rest to be isolated; and he had made regular visits during which he had examined not only the positive cases but also the remainder of the girls.

'Treatment?' I asked.

He shrugged slightly. 'As soon as I got the confirmation from the bacteriologist, I decided that I'd have to lay in a supply of penicillin and take over the school fridges for storage. But the old girl wouldn't hear of it. She thought I was just trying to make things awkward for her and insisted that nothing was to be done until you or some other specialist had been consulted. So all I've done is to keep the poor girls as comfortable as possible by local treatment and leave the rest to your superior judgement – which will, I suppose, be penicillin or some other antibiotic drug of your preference.'

'You're quite right,' I returned, 'which just shows you that people can't recognize a competent doctor when they see one.' His last sentence had suggested mild ruffled feathers, which I thought had better be smoothed. 'You've no line on the causation, I suppose?'

'Not a thing,' he replied, 'and I haven't dared to make any sort of inquiries. The Holiwell would only have come down on me like a ton of bricks, for it was quite clear she was hoping all the time that you would say the whole thing was an attempted frame-up on my part. Though why I should want to ruin her, I don't know. The school's quite a useful little addition to my practice.'

When I went to see Miss Holiwell, I found that the hopes of which Balmer had spoken were still not quite dead.

'I do hope, doctor,' she said, 'that you find the situation is not so black as Dr Balmer has painted it.'

'I wish I could say so,' I answered, 'but there's no getting away from the facts of the case. The bacteriologist's report is quite conclusive as regards gonococcal infection, and one or two of the cases seem to be fairly severe – more so than I had expected. I want to examine all the girls for myself.'

By this time, thanks to Balmer's efforts, medical examination had come to be accepted as a routine, so I had no difficulties. Some of the questions I asked were, I think, a little more searching than they had previously faced, and as a result I isolated three more girls as suspects, bringing the total up to fourteen. I do not know what Miss Holiwell would have thought if there had been two only to make the sum an unlucky thirteen. From these new cases I collected specimens, and then I returned to the headmistress's study to discuss my plan of campaign.

'I take it,' I said, when I had explained my findings to her, 'that you would rather not have the proved cases taken away to the local hospital.'

She shook her head determinedly, 'Certainly not, if it can be avoided,' she replied.

'Very well, then,' I said. 'This is what I propose. I am going to turn the whole school into a hospital for the time being, and I shall arrange for nursing staff to come down here. They will be in complete charge during their presence here – under my direction, of course. The general routine of the school must cease altogether.'

'Is all this necessary?' she asked, with unexpected weakness. She looked quite deflated.

'Yes,' I said. 'I don't believe in taking chances any further where children are concerned, and I think that thoroughgoing measures of this kind will also help you as showing that you were resolved to treat the situation courageously and energetically.'

She smiled and revived a little, as I had intended her to do.

'The first thing is to begin treatment at the earliest opportunity. In gonorrhoeal infections with adults, I use, as a rule, penicillin only, and I am confident that it is sufficient but, as I say, where children are concerned it is necessary to make absolutely sure. I shall therefore combine penicillin injections with sulphonamide treatment – that is what you probably know as 693,' I added in explanation, as she looked a trifle puzzled. 'That concerns the girls in whom the disease has been actually diagnosed. But the matter can't rest there. There may be cases showing no symptoms at all and acting as 'carriers' that is, passing on infection. I propose, therefore, to administer penicillin to every girl in the school.'

'It seems rather drastic,' she said doubtfully.

'Desperate diseases are by desperate remedies cured,' I commented without great originality. 'I'm not saying that vulvo-vaginitis is a desperate disease, and I certainly wouldn't describe penicillin as a desperate remedy – far from it. But I think the general situation warrants it.'

'I'm glad you see it like that, doctor,' she said. 'I place myself entirely in your hands.'

'Very well, then, I will go back to the Clinic and make the necessary arrangements,' I returned. I paused for a moment and then leant forward seriously. 'There is one other thing that I regard as essential.'

'Yes, doctor?' She looked rather alarmed and puzzled.

'We have to trace the source of the infection. These things don't drift about like the common cold,' I pointed out. 'The disease can only be contracted by contact with an infected person or something an infected person has used, such as a towel.'

'Yes, doctor,' she said again, really alarmed now.

'So I regard it as essential that every member of the staff should be examined. I suppose I can't insist, and if anyone wants to refuse she can do so. That unfortunately is the state of affairs today,' I said bitterly. 'At the same time, if the position is explained, I think we would not be entirely unjustified in drawing conclusions from a refusal. When I come tomorrow, I shall ask you to assemble the staff, without a single exception, and I'll talk to them.'

'It seems asking too much, doctor,' she protested. 'It looks as though I am casting aspersions on my staff, and I certainly would not think of doing so.'

'Not at all,' I insisted. 'The responsibility is mine entirely, and I shall point that out to them in my talk. And your only part will be to set an example – to say that as soon as I put the position to you, you gladly consented to examination.'

'But, doctor, this is outrageous!' she flamed. 'I would not think of it.'

'Then,' I interrupted brusquely, 'you are prepared to make it easy for others to refuse and to permit, it may be, an active source of infection to remain in the school, with all the prospects of future trouble?'

She was silent for a while.

'Very well, doctor,' she said at last. 'I see I must do my duty.'

That was the worst hurdle surmounted.

I returned to the Clinic and had an interview with the Director-General. He did not seem pleased at the arrangements I had proposed, but I had expected opposition and was prepared for it. The Maynard Clinic is not organized for dealing with cases outside its walls. However, I put forward a concrete plan that would not unduly deplete the staff of the department, and, after some arguments and with one or two minor modifications, this was accepted. Next day, quite a party set out for the school – four nurses, one of my assistants, and myself. It was, as my assistant, a young but very clever man pointed out, quite a major operation; but I think the nurses looked on it, for all the seriousness of the situation, as a welcome break from their normal routine.

In its main features, vulvo-vaginitis of this kind has a lot in common with gonorrhoea in the adult. There are the same discharges, but the actual inflammation is of a somewhat different kind, owing to the different structure of the tissues in children as compared with adults and also to the absence in the child of certain secretions which commence at puberty. But the cause is identical – the gonococcus, and therefore the lines of treatment are the same. Until the perfection of the later sulphonamide drugs, there were various forms of treatment, some of which are still of value in certain circumstances; but nowadays the chief weapon is the powerful penicillin and the many other antibiotic drugs available, with the dosage modified at the age of the patient, and sometimes with sulphonamide administered additionally – as I proposed in this instance.

The treatment itself was uneventful. The signs and symptoms rapidly cleared, and in a little while the girls had returned to normal. For the next six months, at least, I or my assistant would visit the school to make a routine examination in order to ensure that the infection had cleared up. Vulvovaginitis is a form of gonococcal infection with a fairly high tendency to relapse after apparent cure, and observation is, therefore, of special importance; but I am inclined to believe that the danger of relapse and reinfection is smaller when antibiotic drugs are employed.

Once I had, so to speak, got the medical organization working smoothly in the school itself, I turned to the problem of whence the infection had originated. I do not think that I have had any more trying experience than the talk I had promised to give to the staff. They were all assembled in Miss Holiwell's study, and though it was a large room, it was quite crowded, for everyone was there, from the senior mistress to the kitchenmaid. The presence of so many people at very close quarters was oppressive enough, but the general sense of resentment and opposition was almost frightening. However, I braced myself for the ordeal.

Miss Holiwell did her part nobly, and I salute her for that. She introduced me in a brief speech, telling the audience who I was and why I was there, and then she added:

'Later on, Dr Miles is going to make a proposal to you. It may seem to you a little drastic, but I am sure that after he has talked to you, you will all see the gravity of the situation and realize how important it is that we should all, without exception, accept his advice on our course of conduct. For myself, I am quite convinced that he is perfectly right, and I have had no hesitation in agreeing personally, as I hope and believe all of you will.'

With that to back me, I began my address, which lasted for about twenty minutes, during the course of which I reviewed the position in the school and talked generally of this kind of infection. Finally I made my appeal – to be greeted by a little gasp and then by a stony silence.

After a little while one of the mistresses asked a question.

'Are we bound to submit to this, doctor?' she asked.

'No,' I replied frankly. 'I can do no more than impress on you its importance and also point out the wisdom of examination, both for the sake of the girls and the school and for your own peace of mind.'

'I see,' she said. 'But doesn't it lay us open to terrible suspicions?'

'On the contrary, I think it has just the opposite effect. The position is,' I explained, 'that these girls have come into contact with infection – which must be a person or something used by that person. Moreover, it must be a person very near to them, for the gonococcus soon dies under normal conditions. It can't exist for a considerable period and be distributed through the air, like say, the virus of the influenza. If examination shows that you are free, you are cleared of all suspicions. On the other hand, one of you may have become infected quite unwittingly – it is possible, just possible. In any event, it is vital to find out where the infection lies. It may be – I would even say I think it highly probable – that it does not lie with one of you, but may be due to some external contact. But there is a larger question. The reluctance that some of you feel is due entirely to the case being concerned with venereal disease, because that has moral complications. I ask you to regard it as just the same as any other disease. If there had been an outbreak of typhoid in the school, I do not think you would have had any hesitation in submitting to test to discover whether you were an unconscious carrier of the disease.'

She nodded, and the women fell to talking among themselves. I noticed they divided naturally into two mutually exclusive groups – the mistresses in one and the domestic staff in the other. Not unexpectedly, I encountered, in the end, more resistance from the second groups than from the first. Yet what mattered most was that, in the upshot, they gave their consent. That day I began the examination of five mistresses and nine domestic staff.

It seemed a pretty fruitless effort. I found no signs of the infection. Woman after woman was physically examined and closely questioned, but the results were invariably negative. The prospect of having to trace some outside contact loomed up menacingly before me. It would be very difficult to trace;

but at any rate if I established that the staff was uninfected, at least something would be gained. The school would not be harbouring a focus in its midst from which future damage might result.

But the affair was not unsuccessful. I found the source of infection – and in the quarter where I should have least expected it.

We will call her Joyce. She was one of the younger mistresses – a girl still in her twenties, good looking, with a brilliant career at Somerville behind her (she had taken a First), and described as probably the most popular mistress in the school.

She smiled at me shyly when she came into the room I was using for the examination. It was a small bedroom used for sick girls who had to be confined to bed. When I found some suspicious signs, I found myself rather at a loss for words, and when I told her, as carefully as I could, my suspicions, I thought she was going to faint.

After a short pause to recover, she smiled rather pathetically. She was of the younger generation and she was intelligent; and she took a rational view of the question. That was fortunate. She was one of the few who had raised no objections to examination, which made my discovery all the more tragic. Finally she told me her story.

'I never suspected it,' she said in a low voice. 'Even now I can hardly believe it.'

'I may be wrong,' I said. 'I can't be definite till the bacteriologist had made his report.'

'Of course,' she returned. 'I understand that. But it's possible. I'd better tell you everything. You see, doctor, I'm engaged to be married.' Unconsciously she glanced at the fine diamond ring she wore on her left ring finger. 'My fiancé has been in the Far East for a long time, but a few weeks ago he came home to be posted to another position here in England. Well, I went to meet him, of course, and Miss Holiwell gave me a week off. It was so lovely to see him again that I think we both lost our heads. We spent the week-end together. I'm sure he doesn't know he's got VD – if he has, I mean. That sounds a little confused, but I'm sure you understand. Of course, he may have got it out East. It won't make any difference to me, of course. One can forgive a man anything when he's been through what Ray has.'

I liked her the more for her views. It was refreshing to find so intelligent and reasonable an approach. She was shocked, naturally; but she did not become afflicted with a sense of guilt, nor did she condemn the cause of her infection – if she was infected.

'I will talk to you again,' I said, 'when I have the bacteriological report. Meanwhile I will say nothing.'

'No,' she returned. 'But if it's proved, I would rather see Miss Holiwell myself. She will have to know, and it's better that way.'

Her courage was stimulating, and she needed it all, for the tests were unquestionably positive. She placed herself under my treatment, and she had no difficulty in persuading her fiancé to come and see me. He was stricken with the utmost remorse and filled with self-accusations, but Joyce and I between us managed to make him take a more sensible view. In the job he had in the Far East, he felt lonely and had to seek the company of men like himself who would drown their loneliness and boredom in drink and in the company of women. Most of the time he resisted the temptation, but on one or two occasions he succumbed to the charms of an Eurasian beauty, and who could judge him if he brought back with him one of the inevitable products?

Miss Holiwell, as usual, presented the most difficult problem. As soon as Joyce had seen her, she sent for me.

'This is terrible, doctor,' she said. 'I certainly did not expect you to find that Joyce, of all people, was the guilty person. If it had been one of the kitchen maids it would have been bad enough – but Joyce! And even then I can't see how she gave it to the girls.'

'I have found out the probable explanation,' I said, 'and I will give it to you in the strictest confidence. Soon after Joyce returned from her leave, she went through the dormitories one night and found the little girl Sally crying bitterly. She tried to comfort her. You may remember the day – you had told Sally that morning that her parents were not coming home as early as they expected and so she would have to spend the holidays with you.'

'Yes,' said a very tight-lipped Miss Holiwell.

'Joyce could do nothing to calm her, and in the end she took Sally along to her own bedroom and she slept in her bed. There, I think, is the explanation. Sally was the first case, you remember.'

'She had no right to take one of the girls to her room,' snapped Miss Holiwell.

'Perhaps not. But rules and human compassion are not always good companions,' I returned rather sharply.

'It's altogether scandalous,' said Miss Holiwell acidly. 'Of course Joyce will have to go. I couldn't possibly have a woman like that about the school.'

'I shouldn't be hasty, Miss Holiwell,' I said determinedly. 'If you dismiss Joyce, you are directing attention to her. Moreover you are being grossly unfair. She is a good mistress, and, I believe, very popular with the girls. Her going would raise very many questions.'

'She is an immoral woman,' snapped Miss Holiwell. 'Her presence here would corrupt the girls.'

'Are you sure that is a just judgement?' I demanded. 'Miss Holiwell, I am going to appeal to you. I am going to ask you to do nothing and say nothing till I have cured Joyce and she has had time to recover from the shock. Then she can speak for herself, and we can go into this problem.'

She reflected for a moment or two. 'I will do as you ask, doctor,' she said. 'But it will not make any difference.'

Yet even with Miss Holiwell, second thoughts proved best. A little later I raised the matter again, thinking attack the best way. No one knew I had been treating Joyce, and though there might have been suspicions, the general attitude was that my examinations had drawn a blank. This helped me a lot.

'I have thought it over,' said Miss Holiwell, 'and perhaps you are right, doctor. The least said the sooner mended is quite a good proverb, you know. Joyce tells me she will be leaving to get married soon in any event, and so she had better stay. It is best for the school, which is my chief concern, and its interests override everything else.'

So ended the scandal in the school. Joyce and Raymond are cured now and happy together. It was an interesting and unusual case, but the chief fight, as always, was concerned with moral issues. How different it might have all turned out if Miss Holiwell had hounded Joyce from the school like a moral leper! One life would have been broken, and I think more, for when the children came to understand fully what had happened, they would have acquired a condemnatory attitude to Joyce and their outlook on a great problem of today would have become biased and warped. When I review this case, I feel that my great triumph was not the arrest of the outbreak (which Dr Balmer could have effected as well as me) but my victory in the battle of wits and morality with Miss Barbara Holiwell, MA (Lond.)

Case 12

PHYLLIS

As I have stressed over and over again in these pages, a very large proportion of the tragedies of venereal diseases are caused by ignorance, which range from complete misconceptions of the nature and cause of the infections to inability to recognize small, but significant, symptoms. But there are also tragedies that come through knowledge – from that little knowledge which is proverbially so dangerous a thing.

Everyone has heard the story of the man who read through a medical dictionary and thought himself the victim of each disease in the list as soon as he had learnt of its symptoms – and has chuckled over it. Yet that is not entirely a wasteful or dangerous form of delusion. It is better for a man to take his doubts and difficulties, his suspicions and his anxieties about his health to his doctor, than to delude himself with the over self-confident belief that he knows all and does not need help. Precaution is better than cure; and in no circumstances is the need of investigating any faint suspicion more essential than in connection with venereal diseases. I would rather have a hundred or even a thousand patients come to me with, in reality, no more than a faint fear they might have contracted infection than one bad case of, say, advanced neuro-syphilis, the result of long neglect through over-weening belief that 'it will be all right'. Nor should I consider the time devoted to the hundred or one thousand cases wasted or ill-spent. There is no such thing as over-caution in venereal diseases.

I believe fervently in securing the widest possible dissemination of the facts of venereal disease, seeing in that the most powerful means of checking and diminishing its incidence. At the same time, care must be taken that the facts are understood, for perhaps a badly digested fact is even worse than ignorance – especially when it leads to failure or refusal to be guided by those who have long, specialized experience. That is not to claim infallibility for the expert – which would be both presumptious and very wrong, for a man is free from error: it merely asserts the not unreasonable proposition that practical experience is of the highest value.

In all my practice, one case stands out as a remarkable instance of the effects of fear induced by a little knowledge that was not enough and of theoretical knowledge that had not sufficient practical experience to form a sound basis for it. It was the case of Phyllis.

Phyllis made her entry into my affairs in a manner to which the overworked adjective 'dramatic' is fully applicable. She did not come to me as a patient in the ordinary way, nor was she sent to the Clinic by a general practitioner. Her sponsors were the police; the intermediary who presented me with the background of her case was a most acute progressively minded divisional police-surgeon.

Let there be no misconceptions about Phyllis as the result of this rather unconventional introduction. She was not one of those to whom transactions with the police are a normal incident in the life's work. Certainly she was no infected street-walker whom a patient police-surgeon and court missionary had at last induced to take the course of prudence. On the contrary, she was a highly educated, sensitive minded, and very talented woman in the middle thirties. She earned a fairly remunerative living as a freelance journalist, contributing to the more serious reviews and magazines, and she had also published three novels, which if they had not added materially to her wealth, had done not a little to establish her reputation for her. I happened to have read them all with keen appreciation, so her name was not entirely unknown when she was presented to me. If it is added that she was of middle height, with dark brown hair pleasantly lit by a reddish tinge, hazel eyes, and a rather reflective cast of countenance, the preliminary picture of Phyllis is complete.

Phyllis lived in a small two-roomed flat in a service block of a quiet and respectable kind. One day, the housekeeper, going to her flatlet with a parcel, noticed a strong smell of gas emanating from it. He sniffed carefully, decided that she had left a burner turned on or that the pilot light of the water heater had blown out, and knocked loudly. There was no reply – which struck him as a little curious, for only three-quarters of an hour before he had caught sight of her entering the building. Still, she might have gone out again without his noticing it; he had been kept busy for the last half hour. A little reluctantly, he went away, hoping that his careless tenant would return again in a few minutes.

He kept his eyes open for her for the next quarter of an hour, but there was no sign of her, and he decided he had better enter the flat. If the gas was still escaping it might leak into the neighbouring flatlets and damage would result when someone struck a match. He picked up his bunch of keys and ascended in the lift to the second floor. As he threw open the front door of the flatlet, the smell of gas was almost overpowering, but he did not stop to consider his own safety. The state of affairs was only too plain. The housekeeper had spent the greater part of his life in the Navy and was a man of action. He weighed up the situation and took prompt and effective steps to meet it.

In front of the gas fire, lying on the hearth-rug, was Phyllis. The gas fire, which was a portable one, had been disconnected, and its place at the end of the rubber tube had been taken by a large tin funnel, which was now alongside Phyllis's head. There was only one interpretation: attempted suicide. The housekeeper did not stop to argue that it was a ridiculous idea to think that a woman of her type would attempt to kill herself, he did the right things. Having first thrown open all the windows and turned off the gas, he pulled Phyllis out and carried her along to a little balcony at the end of the corridor. Then, having made her comfortable, he telephoned for the police and an ambulance.

The services arrived together, the police bringing their divisional surgeon with them. He took the appropriate measures and dispatched her to hospital. She had been found only just in time, and the doctors had to fight pretty hard for her life, but in the end he succeeded, and after a day or two she was pronounced fit enough to submit to police questioning.

Her statement was not very informative. All she would say – and she refused to amplify her story to the detective-sergeant who called on her repeatedly – was that she was tired of her life, saw no future for herself and had decided to end it. And she pointed out, with a ruthless logic that, however, the law does not accept, that it was her life, so surely she was entitled to do what she liked with it. Her going would not have embarrassed anyone. She had paid all her debts and put her affairs in order. The only doubts she had had were in connection with the flat. A suicide there would not do the house any good and her landlords had always treated her well. But she could see no other way than gas – which meant her own flat, and she confessed that dying among her own familiar things had a certain sentimental appeal.

This did not satisfy the police. They pointed out to her that some of her statements were ridiculous. She said she had no future; yet that was the time when her reputation as a novelist was fully made and everyone was looking on her as a successful writer of whom much more might be expected. She replied that that was her affair. No amount of questions or suggestions could move her.

At this point, the divisional surgeon, who, like most of his kind today, was a good psychiatrist as well as an expert in forensic medicine, took a hand. She regarded his entry coldly and asked when she was going to be left in peace. If they wanted to charge her with attempted suicide, then let them do so. Dr Melrose (who, incidentally, I had known quite well for a good few years) was not satisfied with her attitude and arguments.

'If you are left in peace,' he pointed out, 'you may do the same thing again – and this time you might not be so lucky.'

'Lucky?' she said scornfully. 'I was damned unlucky.'

'I think you'll get over that,' returned Melrose. 'Later on, you will see the affair in its proper perspective. My guess is that you've something on your mind. Really, I'm here to protect you. There are suggestions floating round that you're not quite normal.'

'Why?' She was still highly scornful. 'Just because I felt that I'd had it and preferred to wind up my affairs? Damn it all, doctor, if my life's not my own, whose is it?'

'But you see, we can't allow that idea to get about,' pointed out Melrose. 'We can't have people doing themselves in on the spur of the moment. Besides, the mere fact that you attempted it indicates that there's something wrong either with your affairs or your own self. The normal, natural instinct of all animal life, man or amoeba, is to preserve its own life, not to destroy it.'

'May be,' snapped Phyllis. 'But there may be some human beings who've outgrown their mere animal instincts and no longer agree that life is as sacred as politicians and moralists keen on procuring supplies of cheap labour and cannon-fodder make out it is. And surely you know, doctor, that Freud has pointed out that there's a death-wish in every human mind alongside the self-preservation instinct, and that it sometimes becomes paramount?'

Her tone was faintly superior. Melrose saw that if it came to a duel of words, he was more than likely to come off second best; he would have to try some other method of approach. He was determined to succeed, for the case interested him as a psychiatrist. Secretly, though not officially, he was inclined to agree with some of her views.

'We shan't get far along that road,' he remarked. 'As for Freud there are few practical psychiatrists who swallow him whole today, you know, and that death-wish postulate is very controversial. I happened to be a practising psychiatrist. That's one reason I'm here.'

'I see,' she commented scathingly. 'You think I'm a nice new guinea-pig to trot along your laboratory bench. How very complimentary of you, Doctor Melrose!'

Melrose smiled. His experience had given him a well-toughened shell, and he was used to that sort of thing. Her nerves were on edge, and she showed signs of hysterical symptoms. Now and again her eyes betrayed a deep-lying, inescapable fear. She was fighting some shadow in her mind, and it was to escape that that she had resorted to the gas tube. The reason for her attempt was not one of the things that normally interest the law, whose mind is perforce somewhat earthy she was not trying to escape the bailiffs or the threat of arrest for misdeeds. Nor was she mad in the legal sense. If she had succeeded and the coroner's verdict had spoken of the balance of her mind being disturbed, that would probably have been quite near the truth.

For the time being, Melrose gave it up – but he was not abandoning the case. To him she was a sick person, and he believed he could help her. He was relying on his experience of hysterics. At the moment she was in a mood of self-isolation and held an aggressive attitude to the world, which she regarded as trying to obtrude itself unnecessarily into her affairs. In all probability, so he argued, that phase would be succeeded by an almost desperate desire to confide in someone, to abrogate the position of self sufficiency, and to find relief from her troubles by throwing them or someone else's shoulders. Melrose's plan was to make as certain as he could that those shoulders would be his.

He made a report that had the desired effect of checking legal proceedings, and he continued to drop in casually on Phyllis. And in the end his plan succeeded. It was not, it may be remarked, without its reactions on himself. At first he had looked on her simply as an interesting case in abnormal psychology; little by little he came to appreciate and respect her as an intelligent personality, whom he was proud to regard as a friend.

Fencing with him had become almost a game with her. She adopted an attitude of defiance the moment she saw him. But he noted how the look of haunting strain about her eyes was growing. He was deeply sorry for her, but he knew better than to comment on it. His best course was to notice without seeming to observe. One word to suggest that he guessed more than he should, and she would become an adversary again.

It was quite late one evening when he called on her. He found her still wearing her outdoor coat, and he apologized for his untimely intrusion.

'Don't apologize,' she said with a nervous smile – he noted

it at once – 'It may shake you to know that I'm pleased to see you.'

'I'm honoured,' he returned, a little nonplussed.

'I've been to a concert at the Albert Hall,' she went on. 'The Sibelius unsettled me – he always does. I feel restless.' She threw her coat on a chair. 'You sit down, and I'll go and make some coffee.'

'Thanks.' He dropped into the big easy chair. 'Might I, as a medical man, suggest that coffee isn't the best thing for a restless mood.'

'Shucks!' she retorted with a grimace. 'I like it. That's far more important.'

In a little while, she returned with a tray bearing a coffee pot, two cups and saucers, and some biscuits.

'Sorry I can't be more lavish,' she said, 'but next time you must warn me in advance.'

'That's all right,' he responded. 'I've dined quite well tonight for a change, and the coffee will do me fine.'

She sipped her drink and nibbled a biscuit with an abstracted air, apparently forgetful of his presence. He could study her without her being aware of it, and he noted the slight nervous tics, the little tremors of the muscles, that told of a state of inward stress. At last she laid aside her cup and shivered. It was early autumn, and not chilly enough to justify a shiver, but he said nothing. He had an almost triumphant feeling that his time had come. In silence he watched her as she struck a match and lighted the gas fire. As the burners popped, she jerked back.

'Gas,' she murmured. 'How easy it seems – and yet how difficult it is!'

She stared at the radiants as they changed from brownish white to glowing red.

Gently, so as not to disturb her, he leant towards her.

'Why don't you tell me all about it?' he asked in a soft voice.

Very slowly she withdrew her gaze from the fire and looked at him.

'Would it help?' she asked. There was no trace of irony or resistance. It was a plain, practical question.

'I think so. A thing like that is more easily borne by two

people than one,' he replied.

She was silent again and he did not interrupt her thoughts. At last, she began to speak in a low, barely audible voice.

'You want to know why I did it,' she said. 'I suppose it does seem inexplicable to you. I seem to have most things, don't I? Enough to live on decently, so that I can buy all the reasonable things I want. Success in my career. A growing reputation. Nice things said about me by the critics – for what that's worth. A comfortable flat.' She glanced about her. 'I'm successful.' She suddenly gritted her teeth. 'It doesn't mean a thing!' she cried.

'You've a lot to be proud of,' said Melrose quietly. 'A good many people, men and women, would gladly exchange their position for yours.'

'Would they?' she exclaimed, resuming her near-whispering tone. 'I suppose they would, but I wonder if they'd like it?'

'Why shouldn't they?'

'Because it's empty!' she almost shouted. 'It's a whited sepulchre, a hollow sham. They can have all my success as a writer if they want it. I'd give it all to be a success as a woman.'

'Aren't you?' he asked. He was withdrawing his personality from the interview, trying to make himself merely an impersonal counterpoint of her thoughts, like, perhaps, the voice of her conscience.

She shook her head violently, despairingly. 'No!' she cried. 'No! I'd rather scrub floors all my life if I could be a woman. I envy them when I see them in the streets, arm in arm with their husbands or their lovers. I envy them their children, even when they're squawling or being sick. When I go shopping, I think I'm only doing it for myself, to gratify my own selfish wishes; not for my man and my children and a real home.'

'Is it really as bad as that?'

'Yes,' she snapped. 'All that and hell as well. Why did they stop me from killing myself? What right had they to condemn me to live?'

She began to weep, copiously, distressingly. Melrose let her cry. It was the best thing to do. And so, between the sobs embroidered with tears, came the story of her tragedy as she saw it.

It began way back in the past of childhood, where so many of life's problems begin, for childhood is the soil that nurtures the roots of most of our miseries, as of our joys, too. She had never known her father. He had died when she was only four years old, and though she sometimes thought she could recall him dimly, she was not sure if it was her own recollection or merely the reflection of things her mother had told her of him. But she did not notice his absence much. She was brilliant at both games and classwork at school, had plenty of friends, and life without a father did not seem a special deprivation to her. Nor did her mother seem to feel his loss very much. She seldom spoke about him, and because she was used to it, Phyllis barely noticed that there was not so much as a portrait of him about the house.

At eighteen she intended to go up to Oxford. Her mother had an income of her own, which was amply sufficient, and she agreed with Phyllis that Oxford was a perfect preparation for the literary career for which the girl had made up her mind. Ever since she could remember she had been writing, editing the school magazine, and even, in her later teens, having little pieces accepted by newspapers and magazines. But the Oxford education was not to be hers. Her mother died, and with her died most of the income. Phyllis had to look after herself, and she obtained a sub position on a newspaper in the provinces.

From that point, she never looked back. Success came to her in almost all she did. She returned to London on a good staff appointment but the atmosphere of newspaper life had never mastered her as it does so many who get into it. She longed to write in a more reflective and serious way than was possible for the modern daily press, and in the end she threw up her position and took to freelancing. Her genius for success did not desert her; she soon had an excellent connection – and with it the time to devote her attention to cultivating her natural inclinations.

She was just on thirty when she met Laurie. He was a rising light of the advertising world, a young man a year or two her senior, who seemed gifted with the same flair for success as she herself possessed. They seemed destined for a happy life together, till quite by accident, a dark shadow fell across her path.

Phyllis had few relations and even with them she barely maintained contact. There was one exception – a cousin of her mother's. And even their dealings were primarily of a business nature, for he was a solicitor who had looked after her mother's affairs and now dealt with hers when the need for legal advice arose. She called on him and told him she was going to get married. He looked at her sharply.

'Congratulations!' he said. 'I hope you'll be very happy.' She could not help noticing that his good wishes had a very formal ring about them. His face wore an expression of slight embarrassment that was uncommon to him. After a pregnant pause, he added: 'I suppose you've ascertained it's quite – er – safe?'

'Safe?' she echoed. 'I don't understand.'

'Didn't your mother ever tell you?' he demanded in genuine astonishment. 'I knew Amy was a bit squeamish and naturally she found it an unpleasant topic, but I shouldn't have thought she'd've kept it entirely from you.'

'Look here, Claud, what are you driving at?' she asked.

'You don't know, then?' He stared at his blotting-pad. 'Well, it isn't a pleasant subject, but I suppose I shall have to tell you as you're so obviously out of your depth. Your mother never told you the truth about your father?'

'Really, I don't follow all this.'

'To put it quite baldly,' said Claud, the solicitor, 'your father died of GPI. Of course it was hushed up, and it didn't appear as that on the death certificate.'

'It can't be true!' she exclaimed in horror. 'It can't!'

'But it is,' he rejoined briefly. 'If you doubt me, you can go and see old Dr Gunter. He's still alive – I saw him only a week or so ago, as a matter of fact. Quite clear in his mind and a marvellous memory for a man of eighty-one. He attended your father. Shall I give you his address?'

'No – No,' she said in a broken voice. 'Please tell me all about it.'

'Well,' said Claud, not very willingly, 'to put it quite bluntly, your father, Phyllis, was no good. We did warn Amy about him, but, of course, she wouldn't listen. Women never do in those circumstances.' He was a lawyer and a little testy, as most lawyers are. 'Marriage didn't reform him, at any rate for long. He went from bad to worse, and if Amy hadn't had that income from the family trust, she'd have been in pretty desperate straits. It was a good job Uncle John tied it up so well, else your father would have run through it, but it was a pity he didn't make a reversion in favour of his daughter's children. I didn't like winding up the trust in favour of a hospital with you having to earn your own living.'

'But tell me about father,' she pleaded desperately. 'I don't want to know about money.'

'Oh, yes,' he resumed. 'About three or four years before you were born, he contracted syphilis. I don't know how, and I never inquired. It was none of my business. He had the good sense to take treatment and they said he was cured. Then you were born, and the doctors, of course, said you were all right, though you'd have to be watched. You never showed anything, so far as I know, and as it appears Amy never mentioned it, I suppose you never did. But so far as your father was concerned, the treatment wasn't successful or else he got it again. That's quite likely. He had a repulsive taste for the worst kind of woman when he was in the mood.' Claud spat the words viciously. 'It developed rapidly and he refused treatment, though I admit he was decent enough to separate from your mother. In the end he died of GPI. A most unsavoury business altogether. For myself I feel he was never cured properly. They tell me the treatment was not so effective thirty years ago or so. So now you know why I asked if you were sure it was safe, this marriage of yours. If you haven't found out, I advise you to do so, unless,' he added with gratuitous savagery, 'you've inherited your father's lack of responsibility.'

'Don't be so beastly, Claud!' she snapped. 'I knew nothing whatever about it. I shall talk it over with Laurie this very evening, and then I shall go to a clinic and be examined. How could you think I could do anything else?'

'I'm sorry, Phyllis,' he apologized contritely. 'I didn't really mean it. But the thought of that man and all the trouble he caused Amy makes me lose my temper.'

'And your sense of decency and proportion,' she retorted.

It was only when she was alone that the full force of the blow struck her. She felt as though she must go mad. It was not her fault. She had not the slightest reason to suspect in the remotest way that she had congenital syphilis. After a cup of tea in a cafe to revive her, she went to a medical bookshop and brought a manual on the venereal diseases, which, hidden behind a newspaper, she read in a park until it was time to go and meet Laurie. The text had not helped her much. So many of the aches and pains she had experienced in the course of her life might be syphilitic, but then also they could so easily be quite innocuous, no more than the normal ills of life.

In her handbag mirror she carefully examined her teeth, but they appeared to her perfectly normal. She looked at her legs, which were extremely well shaped, and though she was in the frame of mind to see almost anything, she could not accuse herself of having sabre-shins or Clutton's knee joints. Wisely she tried to dismiss the subject from her mind and go next day for an examination by a proper doctor. On her way out of the park she threw the book into a litter basket; Laurie would be sure to ask her what she was reading if she had it with her, and it seemed rather a crude way of introducing a delicate subject. Before meeting him, she fortified herself with a drink, for she felt her courage oozing and the thoughts of how Laurie might take the news frightened her.

Laurie hardly came up to standard. He gave vent to a good many generalities of a high-sounding kind about what should or should not be done in such circumstances but he never seemed to regard it a personal problem threatening someone very near to him – and himself as well. Certainly he did not declare that he wanted her anyway. Phyllis, like most writers, affected a detached cynicism and professed a hatred of sob-stuff, but, again like most writers, she was a sentimentalist at heart, and Laurie's indifference depressed her. It intensified the feeling of impending tragedy that had been growing ever since she had left Claud's office.

Next day she set about finding the address of the nearest clinic. First she went to the Post Office, where she knew a list of official addresses was exhibited. Everything seemed to be there – the Food Office, the British Legion, the Maternity Welfare Centre – everything except the VD clinic. Then she remembered that there was a list of addresses in the public lavatory. Apparently that was the only public place at that time in which the list was shown. Her depression deepened. It was not a happy augury of the way in which the diseases were officially regarded.

But at the clinic her drooping spirits revived a little. The atmosphere was friendly, and under the skilled questions of the doctor who examined her, she soon told the whole story. He was cheerfully optimistic.

'You're very wise to come and see me in the circumstances,' he said, 'but I doubt very much whether you've any trouble. However, we will see.'

His physical examination was searching – but revealed nothing. There was not the slightest suspicious sign. Then he took a blood sample pointing out that this was the only sure check. She submitted without reluctance. She was feeling better on results so far of the examination. It was encouraging, and the doctor did nothing to dash her hopes, beyond stressing again that the blood test alone was decisive.

She found herself looking forward eagerly to the next visit when, she now felt certain, she would get her reprieve from worry and doubt. But the shadow that had descended on her deepened. The doctor looked grave and told her that, rather unexpectedly, her Wassermann reaction was positive. The world seemed to tumble about her ears. Of course, she consented at once to treatment. The period was now of the National Health Service and the doctor said that he will get all the penicillin needed free or any other antibiotic drug, should she be allergic to penicillin. In any case, she would be cured – 'cleaned up completely', he put it.

Laurie took the news calmly. He brushed it aside, in fact, and turned to other topics.

It was at the end of the treatment – which lasted for a few weeks – that the fresh blow fell. Her reaction was still positive.

The doctor remained cheerful, and said they must try again. This time he changed from penicillin to a more recent and more powerful drug, and that would work the trick, so the doctor said. It did not. Her reaction remained obstinately positive.

The doctor told her a lot of things she barely understood. She went again and again for tests, others more sensitive than Wassermann reaction, always the same result. When the doctor told her she had little to worry about, she did not believe him. She was incurable. She knew it. The only thing was to have it out with Laurie.

Still he remained calm and high-minded. Of course, he said, the position so far as he was concerned had not altered. He would still like to marry her – this in the tone of a man saying he would 'love to come to dinner, but he was already tied up for that date – perhaps some other time'. That, said Melrose, was how she herself put it. But, went on Laurie, they had the future to consider. There might be children which they had both wanted; and no matter how careful they were something might go wrong. It wouldn't be fair on the unborn (and still unconceived) young, he said. Of course, if the doubts were ever cleared up ... She rose quietly from the park seat on which they had been talking and walked away with a simple 'goodbye'. That was the last she ever saw of Laurie.

'And that's that,' she said bitterly to Melrose, when she finished her story. 'Now you know why I've had it. Now you know why I thought life not worth living – and I still think so. What have I to live for? I lost one man – not that he was much of a loss; I can see that now but I was crazy over him at that time, and I daren't even think of another. Well, am I justified?'

Melrose smiled reassuringly. 'No,' he said.

'No?' she repeated incredulously. 'What is this? Are you going to give me a pep talk and tell me I've a duty to my art and all the rest of it? Or are you going to tell me that when I reach the stage of GPI. I shall have magnificent paranoic visions that'll enable me to write the world's greatest novel? Really, doctor, I thought better of you.'

'If I had any thoughts like that,' replied Melrose

imperturbably, 'I shouldn't dare say them. I said 'no' in answer to your question simply because I feel you're just like a child – you're frightened of a bogey.'

'I think that's more stupid than what I suggested,' she retorted. 'It doesn't even make sense. I'm not quite an ignoramus, you know,' she went on scornfully. 'Look at that shelf.'

Melrose glanced where she pointed. On the shelf was a row of volumes, all of them dealing with venereal diseases. She must have spent a considerable sum of money on acquiring a library that quite a number of doctors would have envied.

'Well?' he asked. 'What about it?'

'Only that I happen to have read the subject up,' she replied.

'And from that you've decided that you're incurable – assuming that you're suffering from congenital syphilis?' he inquired evenly.

She nodded.

'Do you understand all you've read?' he went on.

She looked a little doubtful. 'I wouldn't say that, because there is a lot I'm not interested in, and besides I'm not too well up in medical terms – some of them are so very odd. But I know sufficient to understand that a positive Wassermann reaction means you're infected.'

'I see. Did the clinic doctor tell you that?'

'No-o-o.' She drew out the word. 'Not exactly that. But then he was skating round and round trying to explain away his own failure. You see, I've been treated with the latest and the most potent drugs available and I'm still positive. Therefore my case is hopeless.'

'I'm sorry,' said Melrose, 'but I've got to disagree with you.'

'I didn't know you were a VD specialist,' she said cuttingly. 'I thought you were a police surgeon with a taste for psychiatry – which is why you've wormed all this out of me.'

'I'm not a specialist, but I do happen, as you've observed, to be a doctor, and because of that I claim to know a little more about medicine than you do. One of the cardinal points of medicine you know, is that when a palpable anomaly turns up, like your case, there's something that wants looking into.

It hasn't been done. I'm rather surprised the clinic let you go.'

'They didn't want to,' she said. 'They badgered me to go again and have further treatment, but I didn't see the point of going through with that tragic farce all over again. I'd had enough.'

'Well, my girl, you're going to have some more.'

'I beg your pardon? I didn't know you had the right to give me orders. That's what it sounded like.'

'I didn't mean it quite like that,' he replied, 'though I'm not sure it wouldn't be best to take you by the scruff of your neck and make you do what I'm going to propose.'

'Why should you be interested in me?' she demanded.

'First, because I like you, and I hope you look on me as your friend,' he returned. 'Second, because I'm a bit of an altruist and I hate to see a young and brilliant woman running away from a bogey man and trying to end a life that could be very happy. Third, because, apart from these things, I'm a doctor, and it's my job to give advice on these matters. And fourth,' he concluded, ticking the point off his fingers, 'because I am also the divisional surgeon charged with investigating your case and seeing that you take steps to prevent the occurrence of further attempted unpleasantness.'

'Very imposing,' she commented sarcastically. 'It sounds almost as though you'd rehearsed it. And what is your advice – friend, altruistic doctor, and divisional surgeon?'

'Simply that you come along to the Maynard Clinic and talk to a friend of mine who happened to be director of the VD department, by name Jonathan Miles.'

'And if I refuse?'

'I shall have to alter my opinion of you.'

'Is that supposed to frighten me?'

'No.'

'If I do come, what can he do? I've been to a VD clinic remember.'

'If he says you're incurable, then I'll admit you're right,' said Melrose. 'But I warn you. Don't hope for a cheap victory over me. I understand that he doesn't recognize the word "incurable" in connection with VD except in cases of GPI at their very last gasp.'

'That decides me.' She had become brittle and hard again. 'I'll agree to what you propose, simply because it will be a joy to see you and your miracle-worker knocked off your pedestals.'

He stared straight at her. 'I might almost believe,' he said tensely, 'that you don't want to be cured.'

Her superior smile vanished. She looked, Melrose told me, like a child that had been suddenly and unexpectedly spanked very hard indeed. Tears stood in her eyes and her mouth trembled.

'Don't,' she whispered. 'For God's sake, don't!'

He pressed her hand.

It was late when he left her, but none the less he telephoned me and told me – without consulting my convenience – that he was going to drop in on me the next morning to tell me of an interesting case. I cursed him silently and aloud told him I would be glad to see him. When he had told me his story, with a few dramatic touches, for he loved telling a good story, I took back the curses. I was really glad to see him with such a novelty.

'Bring her along, and I'll see what's to be done,' I said. 'It looks to me as though someone has slipped up somewhere, but we'll soon find out. But my own private view is that this case is more in your line than mine. I won't give you a laugh, though, by airing my amateur morbid psychology on you.'

'In that case,' he rejoined, 'I won't give you my views of the VD position.'

'I'd rather you didn't,' I remarked. 'I prefer to approach cases with an absolutely open mind.'

He chuckled and asked if he could use my telephone to tell Phyllis of the appointment he had made for her with me.

I was quite impressed by Phyllis when I saw her in the flesh. She already seemed like an old friend to me from the detailed account Melrose had given me of her, and I found her even more attractive than his glowing account. She showed no resentment or reluctance, either of which was possible in view of her expressed views. Nor did she demur when I made practical proposals that must have seemed rather unenterprising to her – that she should submit to re-examination at my hands, and, if I thought it desirable, further treatment.

'I'm not suggesting that you didn't have adequate treatment before,' I said. 'Far from it. I have the highest opinion of the clinic to which you went, and I know the people there quite well. But I know you'll understand when I say I can accept nothing on trust. I work only on the results of my own findings – or perhaps I should say the findings of the team I have here, for, of course, I don't claim to be an expert bacteriologist, for example. I could advance theories here and now, but only a fool starts speculating when he's not sure of his facts.

'That sounds too correct to be true,' she said. She had become quite cheerful during the interview. 'It doesn't sound as though you'd be very good fun at a dinner party, Doctor Miles.'

'Perhaps,' I returned, 'if there's good wine about I modify my rules a little.'

The physical examination revealed nothing, which was precisely what I had expected. It was very unlikely that I would notice anything that the clinic had not seen. I had extensive X-ray photographs made of her, and, of course, I collected blood and cerebro-spinal fluid samples for the various tests. When it was over, I told her not to come back for a week. I wanted ample time to study the X-ray photographs.

'Well?' she asked simply after I had greeted her at our second meeting. 'What's the verdict?'

'Wassermann reaction positive,' I replied, equally briefly. 'No other indications whatsoever.'

'I see. And now what?'

'Penicillin – in maximum dosage,' I answered.

'And if it's still positive?' she asked doubtfully. 'I mean, after treatment.'

'We shall know precisely where we stand. I could make a pretty close guess now, but I'm not going to.'

'I shall be amused,' she observed sarcastically, 'to see you trying to explain away a positive Wassermann reaction.'

'We'll hope you won't have the chance,' I replied. 'I've a private ward for you tomorrow. Can you be here about four?'

'I may as well go through with it,' she responded. 'O.K. I'll be here.'

On the completion of the course, I took fresh blood samples for tests in the usual way. She smiled at me when I had finished.

'I haven't any hope,' she said. But though she spoke lightly, I could sense the weariness of spirit beneath.

'Frankly, I haven't much either that they'll be negative. But it won't matter.'

She looked at me and then surprisingly burst into tears.

'I know I asked for it,' she said, between sobs, 'but it's not really a joking matter.'

I patted her on the back. 'No,' I said. 'But I'm not joking.'

She went away looking very puzzled.

The Wassermann test gave a positive reaction. She looked depressed when I told her, for in spite of what she had said I think she was hoping against hope for a different result.

'And what are you going to say about that?' she asked.

'Make yourself comfortable and listen closely,' I advised. 'I'm going to give you a short lecture on serological tests for syphilis – of which Wassermann test is one. Will you listen?'

She nodded.

'You've read some books on the subject, I understand,' I said. 'Is that so?'

Again she nodded.

'Do you think you could explain the Wassermann test to me from memory?'

She shook her head. 'No. I've a general idea of it, that's all, and I know that positive reaction means syphilis and negative doesn't necessarily mean no syphilis, and there's a doubtful result too.'

'That wouldn't take you far,' I remarked. 'So you see, you're a trained and experienced journalist – your job has been to a large extent to report on matters on which you can't claim to be expert, though you're an expert in presentation, and that's the best you can do.'

Her professional pride was touched. 'I could do better than that if I had a book,' she said. 'I'd get it into popular language.'

'No doubt. But even then you wouldn't understand it. Now I don't want you to do anything but listen. I'll start right at the beginning. You see, what you've suffered from is tormenting yourself by possessing a little knowledge that doesn't go far enough. To every rule there's an exception, and they're always the most difficult things to deal with. Unfortunately, in venereal diseases exceptions are very common in all sorts of ways. You happen to be a rather rare type of exception.'

'Is this explaining it away?' she demanded suspiciously. 'I want facts, not words.'

'You're going to get them – predigested so that I hope you'll be able to assimilate them better and not get mental indigestion, which is what you've had up till now. Well, the first thing to grasp about the Wassermann reaction is that it's what we call non-specific. That means, roughly, that we don't use any definitely syphilitic media in it. The antigen – the substance introduced and brought into contact with the blood serum is an extract of animal's heart, usually beef. And because of that it doesn't tell us precisely about syphilis. All we can say is that syphilitic blood produces certain changes – the mixture fixes the complement, which is guinea-pig's serum. Non-syphilitic blood, generally speaking, doesn't; it leaves the complement free. Is that fairly clear?'

'Yes,' she said, with unexpected interest. 'It explains a lot of what I didn't understand before.'

'Good. We're getting on. But just because the reaction is positive it doesn't inevitably indicate the presence of syphilitic infection,' I resumed. 'In certain diseases quite unconnected with syphilis – malaria, for example – there are occasionally positive reactions. Well, you're not malarial and you haven't any of the other diseases, so we won't go further into that. But there are also some indisputably normal and healthy people who also give a positive reaction, and, as I shall hope to prove to you conclusively, you happen to be one of them. They're rare, but not so rare that I hadn't encountered several before in this clinic. In the course of the years, the technique of the Wassermann test has been improved and other, much more sensitive tests have been devised so that the proportion of these so-called false positive tests has tended to increase. It looks, in fact, as though there's a sort of threshold value, and if we could get the test sensitive enough, we should find all blood more or less positive.'

'I don't think I quite see that.'

'Perhaps this will explain it. A man has a small three-valve radio set. He runs the pointer round the dial and says there's nothing on the air but his own local stations. Next door is a man with an expensive multi-valve set. At the time as the first man, he runs his pointer round the dial and he seems to get a station at almost every point on the scale. He says there are lots of stations on the air – simply because his set is sensitive enough to detect them. Roughly, the Wassermann test shows the same sort of thing. Get it?'

'Yes,' she nodded. 'I see now. So really it's not infallible?'

'No,' I said. 'It's extremely valuable. Over a very large number of tests, the proportion of true positive to false positive is so high that we take the test as very, very weighty evidence. It's our old friend the laws of probability. All scientific laws today are expressed in that way. They describe average behaviour. But you can't use them, as a rule, to predict behaviour in individual circumstances!'

'Let's skip probability. I never could grasp it,' she said, passing her hand across her brow.

'Right. I'm not a mathematician anyway,' I returned. 'Here is something that may interest you more. Practically all the animals smaller than man – I mean the warm-blooded animals – give positive reactions. So if a number of human beings do the same thing, it's not exactly surprising, is it?'

She jerked upright in her chair. 'That's astonishing!' she exclaimed. 'Then really the Wassermann test isn't much good?'

'Now don't rush off to the opposite extreme,' I warned her. 'I'm not trying to say the Wassermann test is useless – on the contrary it's one of the most valuable diagnostic aid we have. But it is no more than that. It isn't a magic touchstone. It's impressive evidence, but even the most impressive evidence must be put in its proper place and weighed with other evidence. You see, you accepted the view that the test was infallible, and that's why you got despondent. Not that you need blame yourself unduly. In the past a great many doctors took the same view, and unfortunately some of them still do. By the way, is this book in your library?'

I held up an American work on syphilology.

'Yes,' she replied.

I could not resist a smile. 'You didn't read it very carefully, did you? I asked. 'If you had you'd have seen this, which the author regards as so important that he's put it in italics. This is the passage: "How fallacious is an attitude of staking all in the diagnosis and the evaluation of treatment in syphilis on a single report from the laboratory, no matter how excellent its reputation!"[1] That's more or less what you've been doing. The Wassermann reaction was all you understood – and that not very well – and you didn't take into account the absence of other findings.'

'That's all very fine,' she protested. 'But it doesn't prove I'm one of these freaks.'

'I was expecting something like that,' I observed. 'You don't give in very easily, do you? All right. Now what is the position. We have a positive Wassermann reaction. The most thorough examination of your body, both by myself and previously by an expert doctor, shows no other signs. The closest questioning hasn't brought out a single suspicious symptom from your memory – and I think, as a journalist, you have a good memory. X-ray photographs show a perfectly healthy structure of all your organs. Even the encephalogram gives perfectly normal tracing of your brain functions. There is, it is true, some history of paternal infection – but I shall come to that later.' (She looked surprised at this.) 'Now I need only say that if your alleged syphilis were congenital, it is pretty certain you'd have some stigmata. You haven't. Add to this that you've now had three courses of treatment with most potent drugs available. Don't you agree that, if you surrender your belief that the Wassermann reaction is conclusive despite the lack of all other evidence, you haven't much to stand on?'

[1] *Essentials of Syphilology* by Rudolph H. Kampermeier, AB, MD, Oxford; Blackwell Scientific. Publications, 1944.

'It seems like it,' she said; but there was still a shade of doubt in her voice.

'Then we must go on. I shan't let you go till I've convinced you that you've been barking much too loudly up the wrong tree,' I continued. 'If the Wassermann test is confusing – if it's positive, for example, when everything else suggests it should be negative, as in your case – there are others we can apply. One is the Kahn verification test. Another is the Harrison-Richardson modification of the Wassermann test. I won't go into technical details, because I think you've had enough. I can only say that we've applied both these tests, and they confirm that yours is a non-specific positive reaction. I might put it that your blood's a liar.'

'It all sounds very convincing,' she said thoughtfully. 'But there's one thing that's difficult for me to see. Isn't it rather odd that father should have been syphilitic and I should follow on with this blood reaction?'

'I told you I'd say something about that, because I felt it was a point you'd raise. I've taken steps to investigate it.'

'Oh!' she exclaimed in surprise.

'It's as well to find out everything one can,' I resumed. 'But first I think this was rather an obsession – like the Wassermann test. You took it at its face value, without looking into the facts very closely. My opinion – I'm convinced as far as it's possible to be on the evidence available – is that it is a most unfortunate coincidence. If there hadn't been that history, and you'd discovered you were Wassermann-positive you would have been more ready to listen to the doctor at the public clinic when he tried to tell you something of what I've been telling you now. He did, you know.'

'How do you know?' she demanded. 'He just seemed to be explaining things away to me.'

'Because you'd made up your mind,' I rejoined. 'I sent for the records of your case and saw the doctor. I know him well, as I told you I did.'

'Yes,' she said. 'But what about father?'

'You want it all, don't you?' I said. 'You overlooked one important thing. Your father had syphilis before you were born – quite a little time before. He underwent treatment.

Even thirty years ago, treatment with salvarsan and its derivatives was very, very successful, so I see no reason to doubt he was cured. He died of GPI after you were born – four years or more after. Therefore you assumed that he had had it all the time. But even your solicitor-cousin admitted that his way of life was such that he might easily have contracted it again, and there's no reason why, if he left it untreated, general paresis – GPI – shouldn't set in within a couple of years. It does fairly frequently. Moreover, your mother recognized the danger to you – and she took a precautionary course of treatment when she was pregnant. That's something you didn't know.'

'How did you find out?' she asked in open astonishment.

'A Dr Gunter was mentioned in your story as having attended your father and as being still alive,' I explained. 'I called on your cousin and got his address. He gave me a lot of interesting information, for he has an admirable memory, and he even turned up his old casebooks, which he's preserved. A most interesting old gentleman. The facts are briefly that he himself is convinced that your father was cured at the time of your birth and died from a second infection. You mother never showed any signs of syphilis, but, as I've told you, took no risks so far as you were concerned. You were kept under the closest observation from birth. I don't agree with Dr Gunter when he said that he had to assume you were uninfected unless he had evidence to the contrary, but then he belongs to an older generation. Are you satisfied now?'

She nodded slowly. 'Yes. I've been a silly little fool. I don't know what you must think of me.'

'I think of you as a most interesting and instructive case,' I replied. 'I am grateful for having added to my little store of knowledge of these things. Of course, I'm speaking now as a doctor. As a man, I think of you with affection and respect. All you did was to overrate your own half knowledge to the extent of exalting it above a specialist's opinion. That's very wrong, you know. Of course, specialists trip up – – quite often. But you shouldn't condemn them unheard.'

'No,' she agreed. 'You've been very patient and charming, doctor. I shall never be able to thank you enough.'

'There's no need to,' I said. 'And at any rate you can reflect that it's an ill wind that blows no one any good.'

'Meaning?' she asked.

'You were perhaps a trifle foolish and hotheaded over this business,' I answered, 'but it served to show up in his true colours a man who, I think, would hardly have made you an ideal husband. I hope you won't think that impertinent.'

'Not a bit!' she said. 'I expect I'd have found Laurie out in time anyway, and this is rather an unfortunate way to do it. I only hope he didn't think I tried to commit suicide because I was still pining for him.'

'I shouldn't worry about that.'

The loss of Laurie was, however, not the only piece of good that the ill wind raised from the dust. A few weeks later Melrose came to see me.

'I'm sorry I haven't been along before,' he said, when he had settled himself in my best chair. He always gave the impression that he was installing himself for the day. 'I wanted to talk to you about Phyllis.'

'Oh!' I exclaimed. 'She hasn't begun all over again, has she?'

'Not a bit,' he returned. 'On the contrary, your lecture-room manner overwhelmed her. I'm beginning to think you're not quite the amateur psychiatrist you make yourself out to be. Maybe half your cures are faith cures.' He chuckled. 'Seriously though, it was a grand show. I never thought she'd ever be convinced. I'm quite satisfied myself, and I'm proving it.' He beamed widely.

'How?' I demanded.

'We're going to get married,' he replied. 'And we're not wasting time about it. You must come to the wedding. A month tomorrow. Book it now. It's about time she had someone to look after her.'

'Congratulations,' I said warmly, shaking his hand. 'I'm very glad to hear it. You can spend some of your time giving her a little elementary medical instruction, so that if she must read medical books she won't see them upside down.'

'I'll watch it!' he retorted. 'I don't think she'll make that mistake again.'

It was a happy ending. Yet it began in near tragedy: in this case the tragedy of trying to know too much. Yet though so different from most of my cases, it had one factor in common with very, very many other cases of venereal diseases. The greatest problems were the psychological ones, the barriers of misconceptions and false attitudes. The time has come to bring these into the open where they can be seen the more clearly for the shabby interlopers dressed in frightening warpaint that they are.

AUTHOR'S POSTSCRIPT

In these pages I have taken you for a walk through the wards of Maynard Clinic. I have tried to show you, through actual stories of cases, the way in which the venereal diseases work, the tragedies they can cause, the dangers they contain.

If there is one message underlying this book that I should like to stress, it is that when the shadow of venereal disease falls across a human being's path, it is cast by the hand of tragedy – and it is better to avoid tragedy than to survive it. Yet even when the shadow falls, there is no need for despair, or for loss of hope. It is one of the greatest and most lasting satisfactions that come to a doctor working in this field that he has so very, very rarely to use the word 'incurable' even to himself. And his methods are sure and tested. He has not always to be experimenting with this new technique or that in order to try to find something that rules out the inevitable failures with existing methods.

Jonathan Miles looks always to the future. As he says: 'In my own work I look for a sure method of diagnosis – a means that will enable me to say, after a single examination, whether a patient is infected or not. I look for even more powerful means of killing the disease – especially those that would make an innocent child born with it secure for the rest of its life, which means all its life. In my wilder moments, I hope one day to see an inoculation treatment that will fight the venereal diseases in the same way as vaccination fought – and overcame – smallpox; the same way as inoculation fought and overcame the dreaded infantile paralysis.

These are the things I would wish for in my own little sphere. In the broader field, I would hope that the present mass of inconsistency and confused thought would dispel like the mist after dawn. I would hope for tolerance and understanding in place of condemnation and cruelty, which sometimes amount to persecution. I would wish for sanity and balance in all things.

Some of these are simple wishes. Others are more difficult of realisation. Yet, who, fifty years ago, would have dreamed of penicillin and the other wonderful antibiotic drugs as anything but an unattainable ideal? So it may be that the next generation, knowing through nuclear research more and more about the basis of all matter and energy, may come to regard venereal disease as characteristic of a primitive stage of civilization, something that occurs only infrequently and as an oddity. In much the same way do we today look on bubonic plague, the terror of the Dark and Middle Ages.

And how will this be brought about? These are the steps which Dr Miles thinks should be taken: 'First of all, venereal diseases should be made notifiable whenever and wherever it occurs, and treatment should be made compulsory. It should no longer be left to the whim of an individual (whose reason itself may have been impaired by the disease) to decide whether or not he shall continue to be a menace to the rest of the population. The treatment of established sources of infection and examination and treatment of all known contacts should also be compulsory. This is the greatest and most important single practical step.

'Secondly, all couples, young or old, that intend to get married must by law produce certificates of health which include evidence that they are not or have not suffered from venereal diseases. Only in this way we can assure healthy and normal children.

'The third necessity, wide and far-reaching in its ramifications, can be summed up in the one word 'education'. I use it in the widest possible sense to embrace the school, university, club, radio, television and press. It should be possible for everyone to ascertain all the relevant facts about venereal disease – not a censored selection of them – and they should be able to do so without any sort of secrecy or suggestion that there is something a little disreputable about the whole business. In the same way VD clinics should be openly admitted as essential units in the National Health Service of the same standing as food offices and pre-natal clinics, general hospitals and sewage plants.

'The aim is an enlightened public opinion that can put pressure on those responsible. VD must be recognized as a national danger for which nothing but national mobilization is a sufficient defence. The VD clinic must not be a skeleton in the cupboard, something that once opened is forgotten by decent people.

'Finally I must insist ad nauseam that all this education must be factual and nothing else. It must not be mixed with exhortations on clean living, for clean living is a vague phrase, supercharged with meanings of different colours to different people. Propaganda must be precise and above dispute as to facts; and it must be all the facts. One of the misconceptions to be swept away is that VD is in some mysterious way unclear in itself as nothing else is.'

Jonathan Miles wrote down his case-histories and comments on treatment and public attitude towards VD before the year 1970, and already they seem slightly antiquated and out of date. For 1970 was the year in which Baroness Birk, Chairman of the Health Education Council, introduced her Private Member's Bill.* And incredible as it may now seem, before that anyone trying to stick up a poster prominently on the highways about VD would have been prosecuted and possibly jailed. Anyone unlucky enough to have caught VD then would have had to go through a shameful rigmarole in order to get appropriate treatment that would rid him of his infection. Or more likely, he would have undergone incomplete cure or not have bothered with treatment at all – with all the tragic consequences that this would have entailed. There were, of course, no tracers – sexual sleuths – to sniff out all possible contacts and so preventing the spreading of VD. Thus it was practically impossible to stem its tide. But in 1970 this enlightened Bill was at last introduced and the gates thrown open to sensible,

* Indecent Advertisements (Amendment) Bill

unprejudiced treatment as well as a more adult outlook on the entire range of venereal diseases. The youngsters could now, with this forward-looking attitude, be persuaded to come out boldly and be treated. And only just in time too.

My only hope is that it will not stop here. The new sensible attitude toward VD will progress still further until such time the disease will be wiped out from the face of the earth. If my book has contributed even an infinitesimal part towards this, it would bring me immense pleasure and satisfaction. It would be the reward most desired if not altogether deserved. The credit goes to Doctor Jonathan Miles and his clinic. I am only the mere reporter of his work.